Empowerment through reflection

A guide for practitioners and healthcare teams

Note

Healthcare practice and knowledge are constantly changing and developing as new research and treatments, changes in procedures, drugs and equipment become available.

The editors and publishers have, as far as is possible, taken care to confirm that the information complies with the latest standards of practice and legislation.

Empowerment through reflection

A guide for practitioners and healthcare teams

2nd Edition

edited by

Tony Ghaye and Sue Lillyman

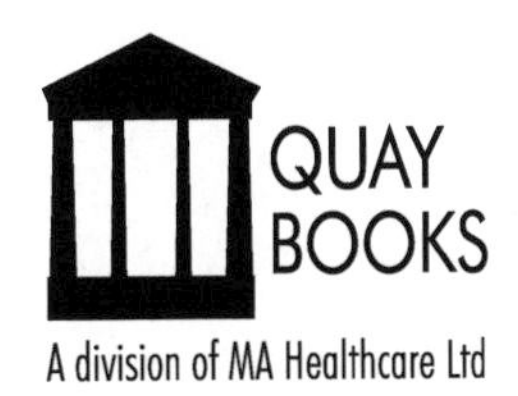

Quay Books Division, MA Healthcare Ltd, St Jude's Church, Dulwich Road, London
SE24 0PB

British Library Cataloguing-in-Publication Data
A catalogue record is available for this book

ISBN-13: 978-1-85642-418-9
ISBN-10: 1-85642-418-9

Edited by Jessica Anderson

Cover design by Claire Majury, Fonthill Creative

Publishing Manager: Andy Escott

Printed by Mimeo, Huntingdon, Cambridgeshire

Contents

List of contributors *vi*
Introduction *ix*
Acknowledgements *xii*

1 Empowerment through reflection:
Is this a case of the emperor's new clothes? 1
Tony Ghaye
2 Ethical reflection: A role for ethics in nursing practice 27
Jan Quallington
3 Taking it on the chin 49
Paul Ward
4 Ageing and empowerment: Questions and dilemmas 65
Ian Stewart-Hamilton
5 Empowerment, participation and rights:
Healthcare conversations with young people 79
Tony Ghaye
6 Empowering people with life-limiting conditions 107
Sue Lillyman and Heather Campbell
7 Empowering students through the use of storyboarding 119
Sue Lillyman and Clare Bennett
8 Empowered teams: Strength through positivity 129
Tony Ghaye

Index 147

List of contributors

Clare Bennett MA, PGCHE, BSc(Hons), DipN, RGN
Senior Lecturer, The Institute of Health and Society, University of Worcester, England
Having undertaken what was then considered a novel approach to nurse education, where theory was undertaken in a higher education setting, Clare qualified as a registered general nurse in 1992. She went on to work in a variety of medical and surgical settings and then commenced a career in infectious diseases, HIV and sexual health, working initially in Romania and then in the UK. Clare then went to become a clinical nurse specialist in immunology. She became a lecturer in 1999 and since this time has worked for Middlesex University, the RCN Distance Learning Institute, the Open University and now the University of Worcester. Clare has also worked for various NHS Trusts throughout this period. Her teaching responsibilities have been with post-registration nurses undertaking degree and masters courses in nursing and pre-registration nursing. Specialist areas of interest for me include learning theory, health promotion, sexual health, HIV and applied leadership studies. She is currently undertaking a Professional Doctorate in Nursing at Cardiff University.

Heather Campbell SRN, NDN, PWT, Cert Ed, BA(Hons), MSc
Independent
Heather is an experienced educationalist who has worked in health and social care education since 1983. She has spent the last 15 years specialising in cancer and palliative care education and practice in a variety of settings the most recent as a Head of Education in a hospice in the West Midlands. Predominant interests include psychosocial and ethical issues. At the present time Heather is preparing for further study hoping to explore the reasons why people care for the dying

Tony Ghaye, Cert Ed, BEd (Hons), MA(Educ), PhD
Professor and Director, Reflective Learning-International, Gloucester, England
In his working life Tony has been fortunate in being able to work with and learn from a very wide range of professionals, including nurses, midwives, health visitors, GPs, social workers, police and probation officers, therapists of various kinds, osteopaths, sports coaches and school teachers. He has also experienced the privilege and challenge of working with individuals and communities in developing countries including emerging nations in East Africa. All this experience

has energised his commitment to inter-professional learning and multi-disciplinary working to help to improve what we do with and for others. Tony sees learning through the practices of reflection as a central part of his work on quality of life issues, personal development and service improvement. He is the founder and editor-in-chief of the multi-professional international journal, *Reflective Practice: International and Multidisciplinary Perspectives*, published by Routledge Taylor and Francis.

Sue Lillyman, MA (Ed), BSc (Nursing), RGN, RM, DPSN, PGCE, (FAHE), RNT
Senior Lecturer, Allied Health Sciences, Institute of Health and Society, University of Worcester, England
Sue is a qualified registered general nurse and midwife. She has clinical experience in various areas of nursing including: intensive care, gynaecology, care of the elderly, rehabilitation and acute and tropical medicine. Sue entered nurse education in 1989. She is currently working at the University of Worcester where she continues to have a passion for developing and enhancing clinical practice through reflection. She is well published in the area and currently involved in introducing and working with colleagues in East Africa to implement reflection and reflective practice into the nursing curricula there.

Jan Quallington, DMed Eth, MA, BEd (Hons 1st class), PG Cert Leadership, RGN
Head of Quality Assurance and Enhancement, Institute of Health and Society, University of Worcester, England
Jan began her career in general nursing, working in acute medicine and cardiothoracic intensive care. The complex decision making and value judgements that this work entailed stimulated a fascination for ethical practice and the use of ethical theory to support value-led behaviour and to guide practice. She completed her MA in medical ethics and law followed by completion of her Professional Doctorate in Medical Ethics for which she researched the moral requirement to involve the public in healthcare decision-making. Her current research interest is focused on ethical leadership and the development of practitioners who are able to reflect purposefully on their practice in order to take personal responsibility to deliver value-based care.

Ian Stuart-Hamilton MA(Oxon), PhD, CPsychol, AFBPsS, FHEA
Professor and Head of Research and External Activity, University of Glamorgan.
Ian's research career has primarily been in gerontology. After an initial period

working jointly for the Institute of Psychiatry and Manchester University's Age Concern Centre on the intellectual effects of Alzheimer's disease, he co-authored an MRC-funded project to examine the effects of ageing on reading and spelling skills. Subsequent to this, Ian has written extensively about the effects of senescent ageing on the performance of traditional Piagetian and other 'childhood' tasks, educational gerontology and on changing images of ageing by both older and younger adults. He is editor/co-editor of two textbooks on ageing and is the sole author of five other textbooks, one of which, *The Psychology of Ageing* (Jessica Kingsley Publishers, 1994), is entering its third edition and has been translated into six languages.

Paul A Ward BA (Hons), DIP Nursing, RMN
Mental Health Nurse, Herefordshire
Having served in the Royal Air Force medical trades, Paul entered work in the NHS in 1987 as a paramedic. He entered psychiatric nursing in 1996 after graduating from Manchester Metropolitan University and University of Worcester, Worcester.

Introduction

Empowerment and opportunities to experience power and control in one's life contribute to health and wellness. Research has demonstrated that health and well-being are intimately tied to and are consequences of power and powerlessness. Powerlessness or lack of control in one's life is a well-known risk factor for disease. Conversely, empowerment and opportunities to experience power and control in one's life contribute to health and wellness (Varkey et al, 2010). Empowerment is a process by which individuals, communities, and organisations gain control over issues that concern them most.

In its widest and most radical sense, empowerment concerns combating oppression and injustice and is a process by which people work together to increase the control they have over events that influence their lives and health. Most definitions accept that empowerment is a complex process and it can occur at an individual, organisational or community level. This implies that empowerment is not only about people changing but also about organisational and system change (Woodall et al, 2010).

One other aspect of empowerment that is central to the 2nd Edition of this book is its link with patient/client care. Arguably, a supportive and patient-centred relationship is, at the very least, an enabling one; at best it is an empowering one. In this context empowerment is related to concepts such as self-efficacy and self-esteem. Here empowerment reflects a type of support that enables and motivates people to take the necessary steps to manage and improve their health in a self-directed manner. Empowerment can therefore be described as being characterised by responsibility and readiness for change.

Some questions that might help patients/clients gauge the nature and extent of 'being empowered' therefore might be:

- How far do you feel in control of your health?
- How far do you know what to do to take care of your health problem?
- How far do you believe that your health problem will improve?
- How far do you advocate more for yourself?
- How far do you have techniques you can use when your symptoms get worse?

In this 2nd Edition there is an underlying position that empowerment is fundamentally based upon the idea that it can be conceived both as a process and an outcome and requires appreciation. Firstly, appreciating what is special and unique about ourselves and those we work with and care for. This casts empowerment in the role of trying to amplify the positive. Secondly, an appreciation of the unexpected and how to respond to this in a positive manner. This casts empowerment in the role of empathising with others and sensitively managing situations as they unfurl. Thirdly, an appreciation that some situations are painful and difficult. This is about empowerment as a strengthening force. What we suggest in this book is that empowerment (in one guise or another) depends upon our capacity and capability to 'show appreciation'.

In this 2nd Edition we embrace the many conceptions of empowerment and explore it richness and diversity.

References

Varkey P, Kureshi S, Lesnick T (2010) Empowerment of women and its association with the health of the community. *Journal of Women's Health* **19**(1): 71–6

Woodall J, Raine G, South J, Warwick-Booth L (2010) *Empowerment and health and well-being: Evidence review.* Centre for Health Promotion Research, Leeds Metropolitan University

Tony Ghaye and Sue Lillyman
September 2011

Acknowledgements

We wish to express our sincere gratitude and thanks for inspiring conversations and significant work in the field of empowerment to: Dr Anita Melander-Wikman and Professor Birgitta Bergvall-Kåreborn Luleå University of Technology, Sweden; Dr Lillemor Lundin-Olsson, Umeå University, Sweden; Dr Xiaohong Peng, Aston University, England; Amanda Chappel, NHS Bristol, England; and Elisabeth Bergdahl, Karolinska Institute, Sweden

Chapter 1

Empowerment through reflection: Is this a case of the emperor's new clothes?

Tony Ghaye

That wonderful children's fairy tale by Hans Christian Andersen called *The emperor's new clothes*, carries with it an unintended, yet important message for those who continue to promote the benefits of reflective practices in healthcare. One proclaimed benefit is that individuals and groups may well become empowered through reflection of one kind or another. In this chapter, I present some of the claims being made about reflective practices. This leads on to a discussion of the way empowerment is associated with the equally slippery notions of power and reality.

Many years ago, there was an emperor who was excessively fond of new clothes. Most of all he loved to show them off. One day, two swindlers came to town masquerading as weavers who could make the most beautiful clothes imaginable. Not only this, but these clothes had the magical quality of becoming invisible to all those who were not fit for the office they held, or who were impossibly dull. The emperor thought that these would be splendid clothes and so ordered some to be made for himself. He thought that by wearing them he would be able to discover those people in his kingdom who were unfit for their posts. He also thought he would be able to tell the wise men from the fools.

The two swindlers pocketed much money in undertaking the work, pretending to weave and yet having nothing of substance on their shuttles. Soon, word spread and everyone came to know the claims being made about the wonderful powers the clothes possessed. Ministers and courtiers came and went. They could see nothing, but they took care not to say so. They did not wish to appear foolish or unfit for their posts. They watched and listened to the swindlers. When they were told to step nearer so that they might more fully appreciate the patterns and colouring in the emperor's new clothes, they did so dutifully and unquestioningly. When the emperor went to see for himself, even he was taken in.

'What,' thought the emperor, 'I see nothing at all! This is terrible! Am I a fool? Am I not fit to be an emperor?'

'Oh, it is beautiful!' he said. 'It has my highest approval.'

And he nodded his satisfaction as he gazed at the empty loom. Nothing would induce him to say that he could not see anything. He was even persuaded to wear the new clothes for the occasion of a great procession which was about to take place.

On the day of the procession, the chamberlains pretended to lift and carry the emperor's cloak as he walked along under a gorgeous canopy. Everyone in the streets shouted, 'How beautiful the emperor's new clothes are! They fit to perfection, and what a splendid cloak!'

Nobody would admit that they could see nothing. No one wanted either to be deemed unfit for their post, or to appear to be a fool.

'But he's got nothing on,' shouted a little boy.

'Oh, listen to the innocent!' said his father.

But then one person whispered to the other what the child had said, 'He's got nothing on! The child says he has nothing on!'

'But he has got nothing on!' all the people cried at last.

The emperor writhed and looked uncomfortable for he knew it was true. But he decided that the procession must go on. So he held his head up prouder than ever. His chamberlains continued to carry aloft the invisible cloak. The two swindlers were made 'gentlemen weavers' and selfishly put all the silk and gold thread into their own pockets.

This story gives us much to reflect upon. It describes different realities and, because of this, gives us some interesting insights into notions of empowerment. It also serves to remind us that it is dangerous to be swept along by any tide of events (including, perhaps, reflective practices) despite loud fanfares and much flag waving; that it can be very dangerous to receive others' 'wisdom' unquestioningly; that we should be able to make up our own minds about the value of things; that we should not be afraid to speak out, to 'go against the flow', to ask for evidence rather than blindly accepting 'reality' as described by others.

There are links with reflection here. Reflective practice continues to gain ground. More and more resources are being devoted to its promotion. Libraries are being filled with texts about it. People's careers are being fashioned by it and conferences proclaim its centrality to improvement and lifelong learning in healthcare work and policy. There is much flag waving and some blind faith. In this chapter I aim to set out some of the claims being made for reflective practices. More particularly, I want to explore some of the claims being made that individuals and groups can become empowered through reflection. 'Empowerment' and 'reflection' are problematic in that they mean different things to different people. They are encountered in different ways. I intend here to focus on views of empowerment, because a whole book in this series (Ghaye and Lillyman 2000) is devoted to the nature of reflection. In this chapter, I want to raise an important issue for your consideration. It is this: despite all the efforts being made to foster empowerment through reflective practices, it remains very much like the emperor's new clothes. We speak about and celebrate it loudly in public and yet we may ask ourselves privately, 'Where is the evidence, from practice, to support such a celebration?' We might have private misgivings. We might ask: 'Why can't I see it when others say they can? Has it really led to some kind of transformation in healthcare? Whose reality is this? Whose reality counts?'

How far are reflective practices 'appealing'? A question of reality

In 1994, James and Clarke set out in a questioning way, what they regarded as the 'appeal' of reflective practice for nursing. For example, they claimed that:

> *Reflection is an integral part of experiential learning and the development of practical knowledge.*
>
> *Much of the attraction of reflective practices is that reflection is firmly grounded in a growing understanding of forms of practical knowledge and of experiential learning. Reflection is central to many theories of experiential learning (Kolb 1984), which is arguably the dominant form of learning in nursing. It is significant in the processes of learning in adults (Knowles 1970, Mezirow 1981) and it is the subject of an influential body of literature (Schön 1983, Benner 1984, Powell 1989). As such, at a fundamental level, models of reflective practice have an appeal because they ground that practice in established theory which can offer practitioners and practitioner educators frameworks in which to operate.*
>
> *Reflection will lead to better practice.*
>
> *Implicit in the status currently being given to reflective practices in nursing, is an accepted view that reflection will lead to better practice and to greater competence. There is, in fact, little or no hard evidence for this assumption although, in time, research evidence may show this assumption to be correct.*
>
> *Reflective practice is necessary for effective nursing.*
>
> *There is an implicit assumption in the justification for adopting a reflective practice model of nursing that reflection is necessary for effective nursing.*

Again, there is no a priori justification for this and the case remains unproven, particularly with regard to reflection in the moral-ethical domain.

Reflective practice will bring universal benefits.

Even if we assume that reflection will produce benefits, it is most likely that not all of them will be equally acceptable to everyone. Improvements through reflection in efficiency at the technical level could be very attractive to those who are accountable in a managerial sense for a nurse's practice. However, the outcomes of reflection at other levels may not be so appealing for that group. Reflection at the moral-ethical level could result in many nurses coming to understand more clearly, through the development of self-knowledge in the emancipatory domain (Habermas 1974), the everyday constraints and limitations placed upon their practice. These nurses could well begin to challenge those whom they see as responsible (that is, their managers) for exerting those constraints and limitations. A parallel issue may arise in the relationship between the student nurse and her or his educator.

All nurses can be reflective practitioners.

Although nurses require particular skills and qualities to become reflective, the message appears to be that all can acquire them. Those who are advocating a reflective practice model of nursing could usefully consider the implications for the profession if the notion that everyone can become a reflective practitioner proves not to be the case.

Reflective practice models enhance professional status.

Reflection and reflective practices may be attractive because they are seen increasingly as a central characteristic of professional action. The emphasis in attempts to define an occupation as a profession has changed in recent years. It has broadened from concerns with the place and role of professions in society to encompass the nature of professional action. As professional practice becomes synonymous with reflective practices (see, for example, Schön 1983), the use of reflective practitioner models of action could have some value in enhancing the professional status of nursing.

Reflective practices value each nurse's professional knowledge.

Implicit in the concept of reflective practices is the valuing of each practitioner's own personal knowledge. As such, reflective practice models of nursing appear to

> *value individual nursing practitioners and the contribution each of them has to offer. Reflective practices are apparently grounded in such 'high-level' values as democracy and equality and may, as a result, pose an attraction for many. A consequence of reflective practices is that nursing knowledge is not possessed by an elite group which has sole access to it; rather, all nurses hold their own theory of nursing. This could well have implications for the way nursing theory is conceptualised and generated.*
>
> (James and Clarke 1994: 82–90)

What are some of the current claims being made for reflective practices? Whose reality? Whose fantasy?

During the last decade reflective practices have continued to gain ground in the hearts, minds and practices of healthcare workers locally, and, in implementing new Government policy, throughout the National Health Service in the UK. There appear to be five broad claims being made for reflective practices. In general, these claims suggest that reflective practices are a good thing, that they make you feel good and that reflective practitioners make a positive difference in the clinical workplace. Some of these claims are more explicitly supported with evidence than others. I want, briefly, to set out the nature of these claims as I have come to understand them in the context of evidence-based practice and professionalism. It is prudent to 'test' the validity of each claim – we should not accept any claim uncritically. By so testing, we might move to a clearer conception of what reflective practices are and are not. I stress the plural term 'reflective practices' (see Ghaye and Lillyman, 2011) as there are many ways to reflect with practice in mind.

Claim 1: Reflective practices improve the quality of the care we give

- We can now more positively claim a link between reflection as personal and collective renewal and regeneration on the one hand, and improvements in the quality of action in practice on the other. For example, we can now find more examples of claims such as 'Reflective practice has transformed the work of ...' (Rushton 1999).
- These improvements can be known, valued and attributed to the processes of reflection-on-action.
- Becoming more reflective is increasingly being linked with the idea that the healthcare professional becomes a better practitioner. This is due to reflective practices forming a more explicit and secure part of our day-to-day work (Ghaye and Lillyman 2000).

Claim 2: Reflective practices enhance individual and collective professional development

- The process of deepening our understanding and extending our professionalism is a consequence of reflecting on our clinical experiences.
- Reflective practices can help the healthcare worker to see more clearly and deeply. In this way, learning through reflection helps to develop confidence and competence. It can give us a greater sense of control over our own work. Some would go further and claim that reflective practices empower us. But what does this mean? Is this an over-claim? Does empowerment mean the confidence and ability to contest current healthcare trends, policies and practices? Does it mean the commitment, energy and capability to work collaboratively with significant others in conceiving, implementing and evaluating the impact of transformative healthcare action at the local, regional and national level? Does empowerment mean being able to describe, explain and justify clinical practice when called upon to do so? Is empowerment through reflection a case of the emperor's new clothes? More about this later.
- Reflective practices can close the gap between what we say and what we do, and between our intentions and our achievements. In so doing, we gain a deeper understanding of the synchronicity and contradictions between our professional values and the workplace practices through which these values are expressed. It is, of course, a very difficult thing to be absolutely consistent. No one healthcare worker or NHS trust ever is. It is difficult not to be a 'living contradiction' (Whitehead 1993).

Claim 3: Reflective practices change the 'power' relationship between academics and practitioners by broadening who generates and controls knowledge for safe and competent healthcare

- Knowledge is not simply acquired from outside, taken on board, transferred and applied to the clinical environment; it is also acquired through critical reflections on practice. We can caricature this process as taking sole power and control away from one group, which we might generally call the academics or 'academy' representing the positivistic-bourgeois research tradition, in order to acknowledge that healthcare practitioners themselves have the power and right to control the processes of knowledge production and consumption.
- In addition to the principal modes through which the nursing profession has historically acquired knowledge – namely through tradition, authority,

borrowing, trial and error, role modelling and mentorship (Ghaye et al 1996), we can now legitimately add another. That is, the personal, practical knowledge acquired through reflective practices. The knowledge generated through reflective practices is knowledge generated to improve the lebenswelt (that is, the world of everyday life).

Claim 4: Reflective practices improve the clinical environment

- Reflective practices may not only improve individual and group work but can also transform the practice area in the medium and long term.
- Reflective practitioners should not ignore the 'structures' which condition their practice. Only by being 'critical' of them can the improvement process take a hold. The structures are embedded in the practical and micro-world of each of us. They are right there in front of us, every day, as we strive to give quality care to make the lives of the sick, aged, mentally ill, disabled and other groups more worthwhile, dignified and fulfilling.

Claim 5: Reflective practices help to build a better world

- Reflective practices not only connect with the 'local', immediate and that which is directly, right now, within our sphere of influence. They can also connect with hopes, intentions and struggles for more just, democratic, compassionate, caring and dignified healthcare systems.

In order for these claims to acquire more acceptance and credibility, there are five areas in which we might place more effort and questioning attention. The first is concerned with recent emphasis on evidence-based practice (McSherry and Haddock 1999). Here we need to be very clear about what we mean by 'evidence', and which evidence is most appropriate to illuminate and resolve particular kinds of problems.

Secondly, and as a consequence of this, we need to clarify the different and fundamental interests and value positions of reflective practices. Who holds them? Where do they come from and why? Are the interests to do with personal renewal and development and/or with producing knowledge which can be applied to practice? Are the interests associated with solving healthcare problems, with understanding the life worlds of healthcare workers and clients and/or to do with organisational change? Are the interests essentially individualistic and private and/or to do with collective workplace learning where:

> *... workplace knowledge production means participation in the praxis of intervention and construction of new ways of working and new working goals, and in the formulation of more complex and sophisticated ways of valuing work, work culture and its place in people's lifeworlds.*
>
> (McTaggart 1994: 320–1)

What other interests might reflective practices serve? There are many. Individual and collective empowerment, for example?

Thirdly, I believe we need to have a much greater discussion about the ontological, epistemological and methodological aspects of the processes of reflective practices within healthcare, and to link these discourses to issues of trustworthiness, authenticity and usefulness.

Fourthly, more attention needs to be given to the nature and potency of the theories-of-action which can arise from reflections on practice. This is not simply a case of trying to make 'theory' more practical, or practice more 'theoretical', with the hope that this will improve healthcare. Our practices and the values they embody need to be made explicit.

Finally, the way reflective practices inter-relate with the notion of collaborative practitioner research needs to be discussed more widely, and shared.

So, how do these claims link to understandings of empowerment? A question of multiple realities

The word 'empowerment' crops up a great deal in healthcare. There is no universally agreed definition of it. As soon as we get into the literature on empowerment we find that it is linked to a number of ideas and expressions. I have space to mention only a few here. These and others are elaborated further throughout this book. Two excellent supporting texts on empowerment are Jack (1995) and Kendall (1998). What follows here are some thumbnail sketches of conceptions of empowerment. Hopefully, they will act to sensitise the reader to the richness of the term and help to frame what comes later. The sketches that follow are not mutually exclusive, but rather overlap and inter-relate.

It means what you want it to mean

I wonder if empowerment is any more than a fancy name for doing a good job as a leader, manager or supervisor, or is an empowerer just an all-round good egg who is always willing to help anyone who needs a bit of support? A concept to make something ordinary sound 'academic' and 'theoretical', or just plain common sense? And does it matter what it means anyway as long as the people who use it know what they mean and how they interpret it in the context of their work (Bell and Harrison 1998: 66)?

Wallcraft (1994) also reminds us that empowerment, like reflection, has many meanings:

> *For some people empowerment may mean having a place on the management committee or the local joint care planning team. Some people may feel empowered by beginning to write poetry or by setting up a self-help group to reduce their dependence on drugs. For some it means getting a good job, going back to college or making new relationships. For others empowerment means ceasing to try to meet the expectations of society and simply living life in their own way at last ... Empowerment is risky, but it is our right as human beings.*
>
> (Wallcraft 1994: 9)

Empowerment, then, can be seen to cover a wide range of activities,

> *... from the power of users to choose what care is provided and how, through involvement and participation in service planning and delivery, to user control of public services.*
>
> (Jack 1995: 14)

Empowerment as a good thing:

> *Throughout much of the literature on empowerment there is an assumption that it is a 'good thing'. Some argue that it is better to be empowered than disempowered. Some say that being empowered is about being more effective, productive, fulfilled and healthier. The claims listed above all relate – to a greater or lesser extent – to this broad conception of empowerment which has been described as a 'myopia of therapeutic good intention'.*
>
> (Jack 1995)

Empowerment of the individual

When associated with the individual, empowerment is often called 'self-empowerment'. This term is linked to ideas of self-care, self-responsibility, self-determination, and personal control and struggle (Kendall, 1998). It is to do with individuals taking control of their circumstances, achieving their personal desires and goals and trying to enhance the quality of their lives (Adams 1990).

Collective empowerment

Going beyond individualism, empowerment is often expressed in terms of relationships between individuals, with issues of group or community empowerment. This is often linked with the idea of an empowering partnership (Tones 1993, Le May 1998) which may occur, for example, in certain nurse–patient relationships. In relation to community empowerment, Tones (1998: 189) raises the question: 'Is an empowered community merely the sum of those empowered individuals who are members of that community?'. He goes on to suggest that a 'sense of community' is a central feature of a healthy, empowered community. He refers to the work of McMillan and Chavis (1986) to help him define the characteristics of a sense of community.

These are:

- Membership – a feeling of belonging.
- Shared emotional connection – a commitment to be together.
- Influence – a sense of mattering.
- Integration and fulfilment of needs – through being a member of the community.

These qualities are worth bearing in mind as we strive to build empowered healthcare teams.

Empowerment as a commodity

Then we have the idea of empowerment as a commodity, bestowed on those without it by those who have it to give. It is a commodity that is given or withheld. If you have it, you are empowered; if not, then you are disempowered. This is a crude and simplistic view, linked to the consumer movement in healthcare in the 1980s and 1990s. If empowerment is seen as something bestowed on healthcare workers and their clients/patients by those people who have it to give, rather than as something personally acquired through struggle and negotiation, then it might be better to regard it as just another form of social control or oppression (Ghaye and Ghaye 1998, Piper and Brown 1998).

Empowerment as a process

In contrast to this, some hold the view of empowerment as a process where, for instance, individuals or groups transform themselves in some beneficial manner. This usually involves some commitment to a 'cause' or a vision. The process is described in many ways and can involve certain strategies or steps. For example, within this conception we find the idea that empowerment is rather like a 'pass-it-on' process. This concept finds expression thus: 'Nurses themselves must first be empowered in order to be able to empower others' (Latter 1998: 24).

Another concept is of the 'give-it-away' process. Again, this finds expression in such phrases as, 'We have to relinquish power, our role as expert, and pass control over to others.' This, of course, is potentially threatening for both parties. We can also find evidence of empowerment described as an 'enablement' process. This view asserts that the process is not so much about giving power away, as about creating opportunities which enable and encourage power to be taken.

Then there is empowerment as 'a process of becoming' (Keiffer 1984). Keiffer describes the empowerment process as having four stages. Firstly, there is an exploratory stage where authority and power structures are de-mystified. It is a kind of reconnaissance stage. Secondly, there is an 'era of advancement', where strategies for action are developed. Thirdly comes an 'era of incorporation' in which the barriers to increased self-determination are confronted. Finally, we have an 'era of commitment', where new knowledge and skills help to create new realities. In an interesting book by Johnson and Redmond (1998), empowerment is described as an 'art' and the pinnacle of employee involvement. The process whereby an organisation moves away from a hierarchical 'command and control' culture towards one of empowerment, is associated with employee 'profit and pain' and a shift in the power matrix. Empowering workers often involves a change in management style and in the culture of the organisation.

Empowerment as a way of thinking

This has been espoused by McDougall (1997). It serves to remind us that empowerment should not be reduced to a series of techniques or methods. It is more fundamental. We can align this to Dewey's (1933) view of reflection which he described as a whole 'way of being'. How we think affects what we do.

Empowerment as using power

Clearly, 'empowerment' means something different to each of those who hold various conceptions of power. Discussions about empowerment inevitably involve notions of the related concept of power – what it is, who has and does not have it, who wants it and cannot get it, who has it and does not want it, and who does what with it. Power is a complex and slippery notion. For some it is about sectional interests, territoriality, giving and gaining ground, about domination and dependence. When these are understood in relation to empowerment, it takes us into the area of social justice (Griffiths 1998). Enhancing justice and becoming more empowered means that we have to understand and alter existing power relations.

Empowerment as developing a voice

Empowerment is also linked to the ways in which people resist, confront and alter the 'structures' which serve to constrain thinking and action in certain healthcare work environments. Empowerment, in this sense, is associated with the critical idea of 'voice'. Voice is the connection between reflection and action. If healthcare workers feel that they are a group upon which power is brought to bear to ensure their compliance and 'domesticity' to prevailing values and routines, then their voice is as one of the oppressed (Ryles 1999). Challenging this hegemony is about developing a voice and making it heard.

This, it can be argued, will be achieved by a commitment to the raising of political consciousness within nurses as a means of not only having them recognise the current nature of their position but also beginning to challenge and change those circumstances (Ryles 1999).

In this sense, 'voice' is used to enable healthcare professionals to resist becoming colonised or domesticated in the service of the status quo. By implication, then, empowerment is concerned with confronting oppression.

Voice is about communication. Being empowered is not simply a process of 'giving a voice'; it is more complicated than this. Here the ideas of Habennas (1977) are helpful. In essence, Habennas argued that power is often exercised through the manipulation and/or distortion of communication. This means that individuals and groups have a different say in what passes for 'reality', for the shared view, the consensus. He also argued that communication was largely directed, not towards reaching agreement, but rather towards the achievement of ends – the ends of those whose interests the communication expresses and reflects. These ends can be achieved through argument, but also through the exercise of power; the power to control agendas, to use knowledge possessed by the privileged few, through authority. This also reflects Lukes' (1974) view about

> *... the way powerful elite groups are able to persuade less powerful groups to hold views or act in ways which are contrary to their own interests.*
>
> (Griffiths 1998: 56)

In the context of the rhetoric of *A first class service: Quality in the new NHS* (Department of Health, 1998) and initiatives such as Clinical Governance, it is critical that we strive to understand whose interests are being served and what are the underlying power structures.

Empowerment as a discourse

Elsewhere, in Ghaye and Lillyman (2011), it is argued that reflective practices need to be understood as a discourse. The same can be said of empowerment. A discourse can be understood as a set of meanings, statements, stories, and so on which produce a particular version of events. Those who share and support a particular view of things, or a particular version of events, can be regarded as a group or a community. The discourse serves to create an identity for the community; it can create a niche or position for its members in relation to other discourse communities and can link them to, or separate them from, other communities. We cannot become part of a group if we do not understand the language the members use or the reasons why they value or interpret events in the way that they do. So

> *... discourse is about more than language. Discourse is about the interplay between language and social relationships, in which some groups are able to achieve dominance for their interests in the way in which the world is defined and acted upon ... Language is a central aspect of discourse through which power is reproduced and communicated.*
>
> (Hugman 1991)

There are many kinds of discourse. For example, in relation to mental health, Tilley et al (1999) refer to the work of Glenister and Tilley (1996), who describe a

> *... dominant 'medical' discourse characterising mental illness, for example schizophrenia, as a long-term disabling illness, a 'social disablement' discourse*

> *locating the primary obstacles to social integration in the environment rather than the person, a 'human rights' discourse focusing on the 'degrading' aspects of mental health care provision and relating social integration to social justice issues, a 'consumerist' discourse reframing the patient or client as a user of services.*
>
> (Tilley et al 1999: 54–5)

There are, of course, many other discourses which are of significance and enlighten healthcare work. For example, from the field of feminist studies there is a growing discourse on the empowerment of women. In all of these discourses there is a need to understand the complex social, historical and political influences which serve to constrain or liberate people and shape their lives. Tilley et al (1999: S8) ask us to be cautious and not unwittingly to 'pitch in with the dominant discourses'. Reflective practices help us to make reasoned decisions about which discourses we value and use. These practices can reveal to us which discourses – and therefore groups – are being privileged and which peripheralised.

Empowerment as a personal reality

I would like to offer a personal view of empowerment which is derived from my interactions with a variety of professionals in health and education, and from my understandings of the literature. I suggest that empowerment is about individuals and groups coming to know, express and critically analyse their own realities and having the commitment, will and power to act to transform these realities to enhance personal and collective well-being, security, satisfaction, capability and working conditions.

This view raises such questions as: Whose reality? Whose fantasy? What power? and Will people have to act in this way? I shall return to this conception of empowerment and substantiate it further in the following sections of this chapter.

Where are some of the roots of empowerment? Realities from afar

I have already suggested that there is a view of empowerment which is associated with the struggle of oppressed individuals and groups for greater dignity and self-determination. This struggle is about becoming more fully ourselves; more valued, respected and fulfilled. Notions of perceived injustice or oppression are almost always linked with the idea of empowerment. If empowerment, in one sense, is about such people as healthcare workers and patients taking action to gain more control over their own lives (Grace 1991), then we have to decide, for example, whether this is a desirable moral and ethical principle; a personal, professional and/or political process.

This view of personal empowerment, of people trying to take more control of themselves and changing their lives for the better (Schafer 1996), is wonderfully illustrated by the work of Paulo Friere (1972, 1974, 1985, 1994), a Brazilian, who is known worldwide as an educator. Reading Friere's work helps us, in a very vivid way, to understand the roots of some of our current thinking about empowerment. His educational theory centres upon the concept of 'progressive education'. This is linked to ideas about education as political practice; to ideas about oppression, competence, utopias and empowerment. His work addresses the impossibility of neutral practice and the virtues, such as humility, tolerance and love, which should shape the practices of the educator.

During a visit to London in 1993, Friere's wife spoke of her husband's work, begun with the illiterate population in northeast Brazil:

> *Paulo Friere has become a political-pedagogue of the oppressed, of all those who wish to re-invent, from the furnace of colonialism, a just and non-eternally dependent society; of all those so-called minorities (women, blacks, homosexuals, migrants, etc.) who need and are willing to participate actively and not marginally, precisely because they have been excluded from the actions of their country and their community; of all those who, suffering from class discrimination, hunger, lack of housing and schools are unable to name the world because society, closed in its privileges, does not permit them to have; to be; to wish; to know. We wish those people, no matter how they are named – excluded, oppressed or proscribed – to have, to be, to wish, to be able to and to know, and therefore to name the world.*
>
> (de Figueiredo-Cowen and Gastaldo 1995: 27)

Reflective practices which seek to empower practitioners owe much to the work and inspiration of Friere, to the practice and experience of 'conscientisation' and the development of 'authentic dialogues' in Latin America. The terms 'conscientisation' and 'dialogue' are central to Friere's thinking and work. Conscientisation

> *... is a process of developing consciousness, but a consciousness that is understood to have the power to transform reality.*
>
> (Taylor 1993: 52)

For Friere, reality is a social construction. This means that we build meanings and construct identities for ourselves within a cultural, historical and political context. We develop a personal reality which is something we perceive, claim to know and believe. It is a reality which we experience and put together ourselves. Personal realities all differ; we all see things differently.

> *Personal realities are... complex, diverse and dynamic.*
> *We speak then of a world of multiple realities, in which each of us constructs our own and has our own way of constructing what we perceive.*
>
> (Chambers 1997: 57)

In any discussion about reality, questions of the following kind must be addressed: What reality? Whose reality? and Whose reality counts? In healthcare, just as there are dominant dialogues (or discourses), for example a medical discourse, so too there are dominant realities which are often top-down, centre-periphery-transferred realities. Sometimes these realities override locally known and owned realities. Sometimes they do not fit and are therefore rejected or become grounds for discontent. The challenging question is: Whose reality constitutes the 'real' and therefore the basis for action?

For Friere, dialogue is a process by and through which we transform and recreate the world. Conscientisation, as a process of becoming more aware of the oppressor and of understanding the means by which oppression is sustained, is fostered by dialogue. It is a means of transforming the oppressed into the liberated. Dialogue is therefore essential for a 'liberating education'. It is a process of coming to know. It is a way of 'revealing a reality' to ourselves and actually 'transforming that reality'. It is, therefore, a potentially creative and liberating process. For Friere,

> *... dialogue is loving, humble, hopeful, trusting and critical ... more simply put ... without dialogue one cannot be human.*
>
> (Taylor 1993: 62)

In his work, Friere reminds us that thinking and dialogue should not be done alone. They move us from the 'I' to the 'we'. There should be a co-participation in the process of initiating and sustaining meaningful and authentic dialogue. If we are deprived of dialogue, we are oppressed. Dialogue is the practice of liberation. It involves critical thinking about the mutually interactive way individuals and society inform and transform each other. In healthcare we have to make important choices between seeing dialogues, of one form or another, as instruments of domination or liberation.

All this is very heady stuff, but it is not 'out there', abstract and irrelevant to the everyday practices of healthcare workers. How can the essence of Friere's work, which argues that exploited, marginalised, vulnerable, disaffected and disempowered people can and should be enabled to express and analyse their own realities and go on to plan and act in ways that transform them, be anything other than central and fundamental to that which we describe as 'caring work'? However, much still needs to be done to join up Frierian thinking and caring work. Much more needs to be done to move from revealing realities to transforming them. This will involve a big shift for many in their understandings of the nature and purposes of reflective practices. Such a shift will reveal the more political and militant face of reflection. Some Frierian principles and processes are surfacing in healthcare. For example, in the excellent text by Johns and Freshwater (1998) we can detect some attempt at linkage being made. The title of the book is *Transforming nursing through reflective practice*. Although there are only two references to the work of Friere in the book, they are significant ones. The first refers to nurses who perceived themselves as an oppressed group within a system which denied them access to higher degrees in the field of nursing (Lumby 1998). The second appears in a discussion of reflection and the development of 'expert' nursing knowledge. Reflection is described as a liberating and empowering process, catalysed by critical thinking and consciousness (Glaze 1998).

> *This ability to become critically conscious is far removed from simply examining an event to see what should be done differently. There is an implicit political dimension, linked to critical awareness, which enables assumptions inherent in ideologies to be challenged.*
>
> (Johns and Freshwater 1998: 152)

How far does empowerment involve reversals in power?

Thus far I have briefly sketched out some of the ways in which empowerment has been described and experienced. I am coming to a point in the discussion where I believe that it is appropriate to suggest again that empowerment is about individuals and groups coming to know, express and analyse critically their own realities as well as having the commitment, will and power to act to transform these realities to enhance personal and collective well-being, security, satisfaction, capability and working conditions.

This view raises the questions: What power? and, Will people have to act in this way? In this view of empowerment, I am espousing the primacy and power of the individual and the group. It is a view that appreciates the power of personal and collective choice and that requires certain reversals in power. It acknowledges that power is 'positioned' historically, socially, politically and also economically.

So, what do we mean when we use the term 'power'? Just like 'empowerment' and 'reflection', 'power' is understood and used in many ways. It is used by us explicitly, and also alluded to in our daily work in relation to a myriad of things, for example, in relation to getting things done, effective leadership, overcoming resistance, managing change, handling conflict, giving rewards, making people feel good or depressed, communicating effectively, team building and working collaboratively. Then, of course, there are well-used expressions such as 'the powerful', 'the powerless', 'knowledge is power' (Smith 1996) and 'power dressing'. We then also have power being used, more or less synonymously, with such words as 'manipulation', 'force', 'coercion' and 'imposition'. But we should remember that exercising power is not a one-way process. For example, when a healthcare group is formed, some members may exercise power by exclusion: some people are in; others are out. The excluded may also exercise power by usurping, challenging or sabotaging the composition and work of the group.

There are also gendered views of power. For example, in Benner (1984), where the author is discussing 'excellence and power in clinical nursing practice', we find:

> *Excellence requires commitment and involvement, but it also requires power. Since caring is central to nursing, then power without excellence is an anathema. I am concerned when I hear nurses say that the very qualities essential to their caring role are the source of their powerlessness in the male-dominated hospital hierarchy. Such a statement disparages feminine qualities and elevates a masculine view of power, one that emphasises competitiveness, domination and control. But to define power or nursing exclusively in traditional masculine or feminine terms is a mistake. The disparagement of feminine perspectives on power is based upon the misguided assumption that feminine values have kept women and nursing subservient, rather than recognising that society's devaluing of and discrimination against women are the sources of the problem.*
>
> (Benner 1984: 207–8)

Griffiths (1998) and Hugman (1991) provide some very helpful frameworks for us to begin to understand the term 'power'. The ways in which power is understood and exercised, and the ways it impacts on individuals and groups are complex. There is space here only to raise some general and relatively easier to understand ideas. Lukes (1974) emphasises the social nature of power and alerts us to a distinction between 'power over' and 'power to act'. These two phrases identify two broad approaches which we can use to aid understanding of power. The first is a view of power as an aspect of social relationships. The second is power as an element of social action. Hugman (1991) suggests that:

> *If power is not an isolated element of social life, but one which interweaves occupational and organisational structures with the actions of professionals, individually and collectively, then it must be examined in terms of the contexts within which the caring professions are structured and operate.*
>
> (Hugman 1991: 38)

He goes on further, suggesting that:

> *... the caring professions cannot be understood without reference to issues of hierarchy, occupation, the clientele, race and gender, which are not isolated from each other in the lived historical world.*
>
> (Hugman 1991: 50)

I shall briefly mention three things here. Firstly, power in relation to the notion of hierarchy. Qualifications and experience create levels, for example as reflected in grades, within healthcare. Seniority can be seen as power and authority over junior staff. Seniority confers power and is a taken-for-granted fact of life for many. When all those in the occupational hierarchy see it this way and do not question it, the power structure is secure and remains intact.

Secondly, power in relation to the notion of occupation. In occupations such as nursing and in the many professions allied to medicine, for example, the occupation represents a power structure within itself. But potent power relationships also exist between occupations. The clearest example of this is the way the medical profession has historically exercised power over nursing and the remedial therapies. In relation to nursing, for example, and a duty of care, the development of a self-confident profession can be seen to be held back by a deep anti-intellectual prejudice attached to women's work in general and to the gendering of skill more particularly. This is where discussions about power get us into deep issues to do with the intellectual and social subordination of those discharging caring work. It invites us to understand the links between power, authority, knowledge production and practice.

Thirdly, we need to understand power as it expresses itself within a context. This reminds us of the interconnectedness of the aspects of power mentioned here. The interconnectedness between social relationships (those involved), social action (what is or is not happening) and the context in which it is embedded. Context has historical, social, political, economic (resource), as well as spatial dimensions. For example, 'connecting' with a patient at a bedside can be understood like this and in relation to the earlier issues of hierarchy, occupation, social class, gender, race, and so on. The understanding of power in a context is beautifully described by Benner (1984). She argues that nurses do have power, although they exert their power from a position of low status in the hierarchy. In examining nursing practice, she describes six 'qualities of power' and names them: transformative power, integrative caring, advocacy, healing power, participative/affirmative power and problem solving.

So, how far can we argue that empowerment involves some reversals in power? I can only briefly sketch in some of the main ideas here (for more detail, see Ghaye and Lillyman 2000). I have presented a view of empowerment as one which describes the way individuals and groups come to know, express and critically analyse their own realities. I have also argued that there are multiple realities which are socially constructed. There are also dominant realities which can stifle, oppress and silence. These realities belong to elite and powerful individuals and groups who impose their reality on others. We can see power as an asset and a means of getting things done. We can also view 'power as a disability' (Chambers 1997). It is held by those who cannot easily be contradicted or corrected. It is a case of 'their word goes'. By imposing their realities and denying those of others, it is often difficult for the 'powerful' to learn.

By implication, 'reversals in power' also involve 'reversals in reality'. We can attempt to achieve this by shifts in orientation (the way we see our caring work), in relationships (how we work with each other) and in activity (what we do). These are not discrete categories, as the following illustrates. For example, I suggest that becoming empowered requires certain reversals in power which involve at least:

- *Developing a more reflective posture.* This requires healthcare professionals to fully embrace both the principles and practices of reflection. Learning and constructing meaningful realities is then about active reflection and reflective action. It is about becoming more aware of how we learn; how this affects what we think, feel and do and how reflection reveals to us how we construct our own reality and distort the realities of others.

- *Questioning transfers of reality*. This involves questioning top-down, outside-in and centre-periphery transfers of healthcare policy and practices. It is questioning such 'truths' as: 'If it is good for them, it must be good for this group', and 'If it works here, then it must work over there, too', and 'If we understand it to mean this, then they will understand it to mean the same thing.' Simple transfers of reality can misfit with local needs, wants and values.
- *Challenging those who dominate from a distance*. This is about listening to and acknowledging the realities of the individual, the particular, the 'grounded' and the local, and not just the realities of senior managers, executives and those in the research 'academy'. This links with the Frierian notions I mentioned earlier of conscientisation and authentic dialogues.
- *Reversals in sources of commitment.* The less power people have in shaping and controlling their professional lives, the less commitment they will have. When senior managers single-handedly define the working conditions and expectations of healthcare professionals, all that employees do is what is expected of them. When tasks, behaviours and performance are defined by 'others' and come from 'elsewhere', and when the value of what we do is defined by outsiders, empowerment, in the way I have described it in this chapter, will not be an authentically-lived experience. Empowerment is about commitments that come from within.
- *Valuing our own practical knowledge and not just the knowledge of others.* One of the most divisive, inhibiting, oppressive and pervasive beliefs in much of healthcare is that the only knowledge worth having and knowing is that which is 'scientific' and propositional in kind. This is knowledge which is derived from randomised control trials, from large samples, and which uses a hypothetico-deductive approach. It is knowledge which claims to be generalisable and universally 'true'. It also carries with it the spurious label of being 'objective' knowledge. It carries with it a sense of 'certainty'. Whilst not denying the value of knowledge of this kind for certain purposes, I do believe that empowerment requires a significant reversal in our usual answer to the question: 'So what knowledge is worth knowing?' Just as reality is ambiguous and uncertain, so too is knowledge. Really worthwhile knowledge can be generated in many ways. We might expect empowered healthcare workers to value and celebrate knowledge which is constructed from the descriptions and explanations they give of their own local practice (Whitehead 1993).
- *By embracing uncertainty and contradiction rather than a standardised, controlled and predictable world.* In healthcare, change is continuous.

> Therefore, realities are multiple and in constant flux. The world has had to adapt itself to a permanence of transitions. We have to work safely and accountably at the edge of chaos (Gleick 1988, Ghaye 1996). Almost everything needs to be permanently provisional. Empowerment enables us to reverse much of our normal thinking about how the world is, how it appears to be and how it should be.

Empowerment and the emperor's new clothes

I began this chapter by retelling the story of the emperor's new clothes. The narrative illuminates many of the golden threads I have used to weave a pattern in words which might serve to clarify the nature of empowerment and how it can be known, experienced and analysed through reflective practices. Centrally, it has been about understanding empowerment through a reflection upon views of power and reality. The ministers, courtiers, chamberlains and all those who cheered on the procession, reflect the disempowered in the emperor's kingdom. Fear of losing their jobs and fear of being seen as fools makes them the oppressed. There are contradictions between what they really see and know and what they say and do. The pressures and expectations which bear down on them trap, enslave and imprison them. Their cheering and shouting serves only to sustain a false and alien reality. It is not their reality, but someone else's. The presence of the small boy in the story is hugely symbolic. He is able to question what is before him. The ability to ask a question serves to break the mould. It is liberating. We have learnt in this chapter that some are more able to ask questions than others; some are more able than others to challenge the status quo; some are more able to ask:

- Whose values matter?
- Whose knowledge counts?
- Whose action?
- Whose interests are being served?
- Whose learning?
- Whose reality?
- Whose empowerment?

References

Adams R (1990) *Self-help, social work and empowerment*. Macmillan, Basingstoke

Bell J, Harrison B (1998) *Leading people: Learning from people*. Open University Press, Milton Keynes

Benner P (1984) *From novice to expert: Excellence and power in clinical nursing practice*. Addison-Wesley, California

Chambers R (1997) *Whose reality counts? Putting the first last*. Intermediate Technology Publication, London

de Figueiredo-Cowen M, Gastaldo D (1995) *Paulo Friere at the Institute*. Institute of Education, University of London, London

Department of Health (1998) *A first class service: Quality in the new NHS*. HMSO, London

Dewey J (1933) *How we think*. Henry Regnery, Chicago

Friere P (1972) *Pedagogy of the oppressed*. Sheed and Ward, London

Friere P (1974) *Education for critical consciousness*. Sheed and Ward, London

Friere P (1985) *The politics of education: Culture, power and liberation*. Bergin and Garvey, South Hadley, MA, USA

Friere P (1994) *Pedagogy of hope*. Continuum, New York

Ghaye T (1996) Critical reflective practice: Towards the big simplicity. In: Ghaye T (ed) *Reflection and action for healthcare professionals: A reader*. Pentaxion Press, Newcastle-upon-Tyne

Ghaye T, Cuthbert S, Danai K et al (1996) *Theory–practice relationships: Reconstructing practice*. Pentaxion Press, Newcastle-Upon-Tyne

Ghaye T, Ghaye K (1998) *Teaching and learning through critical reflective practice*. David Fulton, London

Ghaye T, Lillyman S (2000) *Reflection: Principles and practice for healthcare professionals*. Quay Books, Mark Allen Publishing Ltd, Salisbury

Ghaye T, Lillyman S (2011) *When caring is not enough: Examples of reflection in practice*. Quay Books, London

Glaze J (1998) Reflection and expert nursing knowledge. In: Johns C, Freshwater D (eds) *Transforming nursing through reflective practice*. Blackwell Science, Oxford

Gleick J (1988) *Chaos: Making a new science*. Sphere Books, Penguin Group, London

Glenister D, Tilley S (1996) Discourse, social exclusion and empowerment. *Journal of Psychiatric and Mental Health Nursing* **3**(1): 3–5

Grace V (1991) The marketing of empowerment and the construction of the health consumer; a critique of health promotion. *International Journal of Health Studies* **21**(2): 329–43

Griffiths M (1998) *Educational research for social justice: Getting off the fence*. Open University Press, Milton Keynes

Habermas J (1974) *Theory and practice*. Heinemann, London

Habermas J (1977) Hannah Arendt's communications concept of power. *Sociological Research* **44**(1): 3–24

Hugman R (1991) *Power in caring professions*. Macmillan Press, Basingstoke

Jack R (ed) (1995) *Empowerment in community care*. Chapman and Hall, London

James C, Clarke B (1994) Reflective practice in nursing. Issues and implications for nurse education. *Nurse Education Today* **14**: 8–90

Johns C, Freshwater D (eds) (1998) *Transforming nursing through reflective practice*. Blackwell Science, Oxford

Johnson R, Redmond D (1998) *The art of empowerment*. Pitman Publishing, London

Keiffer C (1984) Citizen empowerment: A developmental perspective. *Prevention in Human Services* **3**: 9–36

Kendall S (1998) *Health and empowerment: Research and practice*. Arnold, London

Knowles M (1970) *The modern practice of adult education: Pedagogy to andragogy*. Cambridge Book Company, Cambridge

Kolb D (1984) *Experiential learning: Experience as a source of learning and development*. Prentice Hall, New Jersey

Latter S (1998) Health promotion in the acute setting; the case for empowering nurses. In: Kendall S (ed) *Health and empowerment: Research and practice*. Arnold, London

Le May A (1998) Communication skills. In: Redfern S, Ross F (eds) *Nursing elderly people*. Harcourt Brace, Edinburgh

Lukes S (1974) *Power: A radical view*. Macmillan, London

Lumby J (1998) Transforming nursing through reflective practice. In: Johns C, Freshwater D (eds) *Transforming nursing through reflective practice*. Blackwell Science, Oxford

McDougall L (1997) Patient empowerment: Fact or fiction? *Mental Health Nursing* 17: 4–5

McMillan D, Chavis D (1986) Sense of community: A definition and theory. *Journal of Community Psychology* **14**: 6–23

McSherry R, Haddock J (1999) Evidence-based health care: Its place within clinical governance. *British Journal of Nursing* **8**(2): 113–7

McTaggart R (1994) Participatory action research. *Educational Action Research Journal* **2**(3): 313–37

Mezirow J (1981) A critical theory of adult learning and adult education. *Adult Education* **32**(1): 3–24

Piper S, Brown P (1998) Psychology as a theoretical foundation for health education in nursing; empowerment or social control? *Nurse Education Today* **18**: 637–41

Powell J (1989) The reflective practitioner in nursing. *Journal of Advanced Nursing* **14**: 824–32

Rushton B (1999) Pause for thought. *Mental Health Care* **2**(8): 277–9

Ryles S (1999) A concept analysis of empowerment: Its relationship to mental health nursing. *Journal of Advanced Nursing* **29**(3): 600–7

Schafer T (1996) Empowering service users: The myth, the reality and the hope. *Journal of Psychiatric and Mental Health Nursing* **3**: 391–4

Schön D (1983) *The reflective practitioner.* Basic Books, New York

Smith J (1996) *Empowering people.* Kogan Page, London

Taylor P (1993) *The texts of Paulo Friere.* Open University Press, Milton Keynes

Tilley S, Pollock L, Tait L (1999) Discourses on empowerment. *Journal of Psychiatric and Mental Health Nursing* **6**: 53–60

Tones K (1993) The theory of health promotion: Implications for nursing. In: Wilson-Barnett J, Macleod C (eds) *Research in health promotion and nursing.* Macmillan, Basingstoke

Tones K (1998) Empowerment for health: The challenge. In: Kendall S (ed) *Health and empowerment: Research and practice.* Arnold, London

Wallcraft J (1994) Empowering empowerment: Professionals and self-advocacy projects. *Mental Health Nursing* **1**(2): 6–9

Whitehead J (1993) *The growth of educational knowledge: Creating your own living educational theories.* Hyde Publications, Bournemouth

Chapter 2

Ethical reflection: A role for ethics in nursing practice

Jan Quallington

Introduction

Ten years on since writing the first edition of this chapter the importance of ethical reflection in healthcare education, professional development and care practice has become more essential than ever before. The publication of reports that illustrate poor and sometimes lamentable standards of care (Ombudsman's Report, House of Commons 2011, CQC Reports on Care Standards 2011) suggest that care provision is in crisis and that some professionals and other care practitioners are failing in their duty to deliver professionally acceptable and publicly expected standards of care. It can be argued that stories of care scandals in the media are not a new phenomenon. It can also be argued that only bad news becomes news; the countless examples of good care going unreported. However, it is also a fact that public confidence in the beneficence of care professionals has been severely dented in recent years; events at Bristol Royal Infirmary, Liverpool Children's Hospital, the Harold Shipman scandal and the North Staffordshire Inquiry into standards of care, illustrate that not all patients are receiving the standards of care that they should be entitled to.

If public confidence is to be restored, professionals must be able to demonstrate to the public that these incidents are the exception and that most practitioners are providing a service that is 'caring' and of a consistently good quality. In order to do this it is essential that individual care professionals take time to reflect on the care that they provide; to re-examine the duties and values which underpin their care. They need to try to understand what impacts negatively on their ability to provide care and what causes them to compromise those values and duties and subsequently the care they provide. They then need to identify strategies to overcome these negative impacts. Ethical care becomes the duty of all care practitioners as soon as they enter into any kind of care or therapeutic relationship with a patient. Ethical reflection encourages practitioners to reflect on care both from a technical perspective, that is, to analyse evidence and select an appropriate intervention, it also requires practitioners to reflect on the nature of that intervention and to ensure that the values underpinning its delivery uphold principles and values of good care delivery.

Nurses, and other health professionals, find themselves working in complex, dynamic environments in which the nature of service delivery is constantly changing. The underpinning philosophy of healthcare in Britain has developed around the notions of healthcare provision as a 'moral endeavour' (Seedhouse 1998) and a universal entitlement. That means that not only are the public entitled to receive care but that there is a corresponding duty placed on someone else to provide that care to a good standard. In recent years there has been a subtle shift in health policy from a service-focused model of care delivery with the professional taking the 'expert helper' role and the patient assuming a role of grateful recipient, towards a model that is increasingly driven by business values. The focus of health organisations has, of necessity, become dominated by concerns of costs and value for money; decisions are driven by imperatives to achieve efficiency targets and goals that meet external measures and public satisfaction. The role of the patient has also changed towards a role that requires them to assume more responsibility for their health and to be involved both in their own care and also decisions about the type and nature of services provided. There is a danger that in a more cost-efficient and externally controlled service that core values will be compromised, and practitioners need to be alert to this risk by reflecting on practice.

As a means of addressing public concerns about care services the Government has sought to implement a range of strategies to reassure the public. A number of Public Inquiries have been held, whose aim is to identify the cause of major failures in public services and implement recommendations to ensure that similar things can never happen again. Whilst they may have their place in seeking satisfaction for victims of organisational failure, the outcomes tend to result in over-regulation, which is problematic, because it undermines the personal ability and responsibility of individuals to make independent, professional judgements which can take account of the specific circumstances of a situation. Additionally, inquiries can further undermine public confidence as the media reporting of failures and the assigning of blame may suggest to the public that such failures are more widespread than they really are. The benefits of inquiries tend to be in raising awareness about issues that concern the public and which professionals should be able to use as a stimulus for reflecting on their own practice.

Another method that Government has introduced to address failures in practice has been the regulation of values underpinning care through the introduction of National Service Frameworks and Standards and Care Benchmarks, such as are articulated in the Essence of Care (Department of Health 2003), and more recently in the Essential Standards of Quality and Safety, articulated in the Health and Social Care Act (2008) and regulated by the Care Qualities

Commission (Regulations 2010). Whilst the values and standards articulated in these Government documents are laudable and do provide standards against which regulators and the public can judge care provision, the standards are limited in scope and in their ability to secure universally good, value-based care. Significantly, the standards are operated through external inspection and are measured and monitored in terms of provider compliance.

Compliance is most easily measured through assessing component parts of care on a given day and does not necessarily measure the activity of care as a whole, nor the attitude with which the activity was carried out. A paradoxical outcome of quality initiatives that are driven primarily by external inspection and organisational needs is that 'caring' behaviours seem to be affected negatively. A study by Pearcey (2010: 53) suggested that nurses working in the current health economy report that organisation imperatives mean that practitioners perceive that they have 'little time left to care'. The respondents in a similar study identify that 'caring' is not highly valued by the organisation that gives primacy to achievement of measurable standards and other activities (Peter et al 2004).

If these studies, and the apparent increasing importance of external regulation and inspection, depict reality in care services today it suggests a service in which professionals and practitioners are driven to demonstrate compliance without really engaging and owning the values that underpin it. Even if these organisational drives have a moral foundation, work by Grosenick (1994) into organisational failure in healthcare, demonstrates that strong moral corporate leadership on its own is unable to support a morally good organisational culture and that deviant behaviours will persist in organisations that do not share strong moral values throughout all levels. He identifies that shared values and ethics are essential to developing an effective organisational culture and in developing positive organisational performance.

Ethical behaviour supported by ethical reflection of all practitioners is, therefore, important. This not only enables practitioners to reflect independently on their own practice but also facilitates reflection on practice within teams and within the wider organisational culture to ensure that these are consistent and shared. Additionally, given the increasing primacy of public and patient participation in care services there should be a role for the public to be involved in reflecting on professional values alongside professionals to ensure that these are not out of step with public expectations.

Ethical reflection is a model for assisting practitioners to retain control over the decisions and standards of their own practice. It provides a vehicle for practitioners to think reflectively about the duties that are required of them in their roles and to think about the nature and standards of care that they should provide and to which people in receipt of their care are entitled. It may also provide practitioners with the opportunity to identify less good care and the impetus to challenge poor care and poor organisational leadership which often results in poor care.

Healthcare practice, and particularly nursing, has always been characterised as a 'caring' role. Caring is heavily imbued with moral connotations. The notion implies a role for which practitioners must not only be technically competent but also ethically intelligent; that is, to carry out the work in a way that is compassionate and value based and appropriately responsive. Studies by Pearcey (2010) and Milton-Wildey and O'Brien (2007) indicate that it is the caring aspect of the role that is being compromised in the new health business context. This is summed up by one respondent's observation 'caring – it's the little things we are not supposed to do any more' (Pearcey 2010: 53). Interestingly, in Pearcey's study the respondents suggest that caring has been eroded because of lack of time. I, along with Pearcey (2010), would argue that value-based caring does not necessarily take more time but it does require practitioners to engage individually and personally with each patient and to reflect on the way that they should approach care for each individual. In a culture that is focused on through-put of patients and collation and generation of evidence to demonstrate that particular activities have been undertaken, it is easy to see how caring can be marginalised as staff struggle to fulfil requirements.

The recent reports by both the Ombudsman (House of Commons 2011) and the Care Quality Commission (CQC 2011) do not reflect the entirety of care but such examples do suggest that 'all is not well' in healthcare and they should be a wake-up call to both practitioners and managers to reflect on what is really important in care provision and how this can best be protected.

Ethics is fundamental to good nursing practice. All nursing curricula have an ethics theme and students of nursing are encouraged to study normative ethical theories in order to facilitate debates about the complex dilemmas inherent in healthcare. This is, of course, a necessary pursuit but ethics is not merely a cognitive activity restricted to the hypothetical; ethics has a very real contribution to make to practice. Ethics, like reflection, has at times earned itself the unjust reputation of navel gazing. Being a branch of philosophy it perhaps conjures up pictures of deep contemplation on the often insoluble questions of life. Professional ethics does inevitably have a contemplative component. However, its real purpose must be with the practical application to which this contemplation can be put. Ethics is only of value if it helps to inform and improve our practice. Professional caring is what nurses do. Caring, described by Leininger (1988) as 'the central and unifying domain for the body of knowledge and the practices of nursing' has been the subject of a great deal of academic discussion and analysis. Caring has been researched, defined, deconstructed, analysed and critiqued. Distinctions have been drawn between caring about and caring for and about the roles of caregivers and care recipients (Tronto 2001). However, the dominant features emerging from this body of evidence is that caring is about personal interaction with other humans, it encompasses notions of empathy, compassion and ethical competence which must accompany skilled technical competence.

Caring, because of its intimate involvement with others, is by its very nature an ethical enterprise. In order to care ethically it is necessary to reflect on the personal and professional values that we hold. These values directly influence our ethical reasoning, and consequently the actions that derive from that reasoning, both consciously and unconsciously. Ethical reflection, that is reflecting on practice using ethical frameworks and values to guide deliberation, should be a foundation stone for nursing practice. It is the key to excellence in practice.

In this chapter I review how a group of nurses perceives and utilises ethics in practice; I illustrate through a small selection of nurses' stories a wider remit for nursing ethics that is both proactive and empowering. Studies of nurses' perceptions of ethics and ethical decision making (De Wolf 1989, Erlen and Frost 1991, Holly 1993) indicate that ethics in nursing practice is frequently seen by nurses as a negative experience, invoking feelings of distress, frustration and disempowerment. If this profile of nurses' experiences of ethics is accurate, it is perhaps difficult to imagine that ethics can be used as a vehicle either to empower nurses or to enhance nursing practice. In the light of studies of the 1980s and early 1990s on ethical decision making in nurses (Gilligan 1982, Yarling and McElmurray 1985, Gaul 1987, Husted and Husted 1991), I undertook a small qualitative study to review the current status of ethical decision making in nursing and how this affected the nurses' sense of personal control. Whilst this study was conducted 10 years ago the issues that these stories raise are not dissimilar from those experienced by nurses in 2011; although recently nurses have told me that financial constraints, time and external regulation have a greater impact on their ability to provide high quality care than do the roles of their clinical colleagues which was the case when the original study was conducted.

The study

In this study I interviewed a convenient sample of 20 registered general nurses, all working in an acute, adult general ward environment in one district general hospital. All the participants were volunteers, were female and had been qualified for a minimum of one year. Eight of the group had received some formal ethical instruction in their first level nurse education programme. The semi-structured interviews were conducted in the hospital informed by grounded theory (Glaser and Strauss 1967). This approach was selected in order to prompt participants to relate their own ethical experiences and understanding of ethical issues, rather than to rely on responses to hypothetical situations which might impose my own perception of ethics on the respondents. Ethical approval to undertake the study was sought and granted. All participants were volunteers, were assured confidentiality and were reminded that they could withdraw from the study at any time. Participants were offered the opportunity to review interview transcripts and comment on interpretation of data.

The interviews were structured around five main questions which had been identified by reviewing previous studies and by conducting a small pilot study of six participants.

- What types of ethical decision had the participants taken part in in the previous two months?
- How had they identified that these were ethical decisions?
- What role had they played?
- What strategies had they used to inform their decision making?
- How satisfied were they with their role?

The data were collected and analysed to identify common themes. Analysis of the interviews revealed several themes:

- Ethical issues are the 'big' dilemmas of healthcare.
- Ethics is felt rather than thought.
- Opportunities to take an active role are restricted.
- Decision making relies heavily on intuition.
- The structure in an acute care environment is disempowering.

Ethics are the big issues in care

When asked what ethical situations they had been involved with in the last two months, participants consistently related stories about the 'big' dilemmas of healthcare.

One nurse talked about the discomfort she felt over the decision not to hydrate a patient who had had a dense stroke:

I knew he would probably die but somehow we didn't give him a chance. He was 74 – that's not particularly old these days. The policy is to wait and see if there is any likelihood of recovery before any active treatment is commenced in these cases, but how are you supposed to recover if nobody gives you any fluids or food? It's very hard trying to explain to the relatives why no treatment has been started. I don't feel the doctors understand what it's like having to make excuses about decisions that are nothing to do with you.

Another nurse related this story:

We had a man in for an oesophagoscopy, unfortunately he suffered a ruptured oesophagus as a result of the investigation. He became very unwell and eventually ended up being ventilated. He was a Jehovah's Witness and his family made it clear that he should not receive a blood transfusion. This was respected, although it made his management much more difficult. The doctors did their best to try to persuade the family to change their mind. It was awful watching someone so ill when we had the power to help him.

The issues that nurses chose to relate were all big life or death dilemmas; situations in which the agent is forced to select the least worst option. Nearly all of the issues cited revolved around questions of life and death. I suspect that if this study were repeated today that some issues would be similar but I suspect nurses in current practice are exercised more by external pressures on their day-to-day work and competing interests that conflict with their ability to undertake their role in the way that they would like. Milton-Wilday and O'Brien (2007) suggest that nurses are very concerned about standards of care, that they know what the standards should be but feel powerless in their working context that is cost and efficiency driven to implement these standards to their satisfaction.

In the original study questions about whether or not to resuscitate patients were cited by several nurses. None of the nurses in the study identified more everyday nursing activities as being ethical issues. A possible explanation for this apparent lack of recognition of ethics in day-to-day nursing practice is that decisions of day-to-day care are often perceived by the competent practitioner as being unproblematic. It could be argued that these practitioners are demonstrating the skills of expert care as described by Benner (1984) – that is, actions and decisions are based on experience and intuition. However, it could not be determined from this study if this is the case. It could equally be argued from this evidence that nurses are not addressing the issues of ethics in everyday nursing practice. More recent evidence suggests that efficiency savings in care delivery, increasing regulation, and audit have a significant impact on workload and the way in which professionals carry out their roles and attempt to integrate new expectations on their time (Lipsky 2010). These factors and the lack of a strong ethical organisational culture may be key factors in inhibiting nurses' ability to exercise personal, professional agency and decision making and to maintain high ethical standards. This disempowerment inevitably gives rise to nurses feeling dissonance between what they do and what they feel they should do.

Ethics is felt rather than thought

It was evident through the interviews that ethical situations were recognised because of the feelings that they engendered – negative feelings of discomfort, anxiety and confusion:

> *You know something is an ethical incident because you feel uncomfortable about the way things are going, it preys on your mind... You just feel that something is wrong.*

Other nurses cited internal conflict and 'just not knowing what to do' as identifiers of ethical situations. This was in keeping with findings from De Wolf (1989) who listed the following factors as being the key identifiers of ethical issues:

- Emotional reaction.
- Perceived time constraints.
- Personalising the situation.
- Communication failure.
- Disagreement about what constitutes right action.

Ethics is, as it is perceived by these participants, clearly a highly emotive issue.

Although feelings and intuitions are clearly very important influences, they are not always an accurate perception of things as they are in reality. They are likely to be influenced by our underlying personal and professional values, past experiences which may, or may not, be positive, and perhaps by our own personal histories or prejudices. Consequently, it may be necessary to review these feelings using reflective techniques in order to attempt to validate them. Deconstructing the feelings and events, reviewing them objectively as if through the eyes of a stranger, may more accurately assist the individual to see the real issues. Application of ethical theories can be of great benefit to help nurses to critically examine a variety of possible options. The added benefit of this is that it provides justifications for preferred choices. By decontextualising the issue it may be possible to identify more clearly what ought to be, and why. This is not to say, however, that all ethical questions can or should be solved by the application of pure rationalist arguments unencumbered by emotion. That would be to reduce the human state to that of the machine. Each situation will have its own individual context which needs to be added to the equation in order for the most appropriate solution to be found. Ethics is not an exact science and there are frequently several 'rights' and sometimes no 'rights' in any given situation. To make a decision without taking account of both rationalist and emotive perspectives would be to make an artificial and inappropriate decision. Clearly, a key feature must be to understand and be able to justify why a particular choice has been made.

Interestingly, all participants in this study identified feelings as being the predominant indicator of ethics, yet ethics is still largely taught as a dispassionate discipline when the affective domain is clearly very dominant. This approach is obviously inadequate and is destined to leave the ethical agent feeling dissatisfied and with a sense that some vital component is missing. This certainly raises issues for how ethics is taught and what situations are focused upon. There is a growing body of knowledge relating to the ethics of care and feminist ethics that argues for the need to undertake ethical analysis from a 'situated' position. That is, one that takes account of the specific peculiarities of the issue under debate as well as examining the issue drawing on normative ethical principles. This allows the practitioner to examine what would be a consistent and appropriate moral approach for any given problem and then to apply the individual characteristics of a situation in order to assess whether or not this has any significant impact on the morality of the decision in this case.

What opportunities were there to take an active role?

Nurses in the study felt that their input into ethical decision making was restricted by the hierarchical structure that still exists in general hospitals. The nurses in the study felt that they were generally excluded from the process. Participants felt unable to contribute to ethical decision making and identified doctors as still taking the dominant role. These findings were similar to previous studies in this area (Yarling and McElmurray 1985, Ketefian 1989). This inevitably generated feelings of frustration and disempowerment and resulted in comments such as:

> *We are not consulted, ... in fact I doubt whether ethics even comes into the equation, they just think they know best ...*

None of the participants identified the patient as having a key role. Although this perspective was not pursued in the interviews it is not surprising, given the hierarchy that still persists in an acute hospital.

This perceived lack of involvement reflected the nature of the decisions that nurses identified as ethical and which more naturally fall within the responsibilities of the medical staff.

What strategies were used to make ethical decisions?

In spite of identifying that they did encounter ethical situations in their practice, none of the nurses articulated a consistent strategy that they used in order to attempt to resolve the issues they faced. Listening to the responses it was evident that the participants relied heavily on intuition; a gut response to ascertain the rightness or wrongness of a situation.

> *It is important to talk to your colleagues, but often you just know what is right because you know your patient.*

This response is representative of the feelings expressed by the other participants in the study.

None of the respondents interviewed made reference to the application of universal ethical principles and rational decision-making models. This could be due to a lack of knowledge of theoretical ethics, although eight of the sample had had some ethical teaching in their initial pre-registration education. Gilligan (1982) argued that women make ethical decisions differently from men and would be unlikely to use normative ethical theories and principles as the basis for their decision making, relying much more heavily on those intuitive and emotive responses described by the participants in the study. All the respondents in this study were women. Kuhse et al (1993) has more recently argued that differences in decision making have more to do with occupation than gender and are partly a result of the education and training that influence the implementation of the process.

A second point that should be made in the light of the response quoted above is that it is often assumed by nurses that, as the professionals who spend the most time with the patients, they are, therefore, the professionals who know them best. This may be true but may equally be an inaccurate perception. It is possible to be with someone for very long periods of time and never to get beyond the superficial; it is also possible to have a very short-lived but intense relationship with another individual. As a key member of the team, the nurse needs to be involved and probably has an extremely valuable contribution to make to ethical decisions. However, it is not necessarily on the basis of superior knowledge of the individual but rather on the basis of different knowledge. Most of us, even in quite extreme circumstances, show only those things about ourselves that we wish others to see. Presuming that we know what is best for others may be a dangerous road to tread. Yes, nurses have a contribution to make to big decisions but this is not an exclusive contribution. Collaboration between professionals, the patient and relevant others ought to be the preferred standard.

Active participation is inhibited

Participants identified the current hierarchical structure within acute care as inhibiting their involvement in ethical decision making. One nurse cited the need to be 'manipulative' in order to have her voice heard. Doctors' confidence in decision making may be a direct result of the style of education they receive which forces them into situations in which they have to make difficult decisions, and then take responsibility for those decisions. The experience of complex clinical decision making could lead one to suppose that doctors are better equipped to make ethical decisions than are nurses, although this does not necessarily follow. Critical decision making is increasingly being featured in nursing curricula and it will be interesting to see how this impacts upon practice in the coming years. In addition, nurses need to be able to articulate their views more clearly to other professionals; no matter how right you are, it is not enough to say: 'I just feel this is right'. Justification for decisions is essential and is endorsed by the Nursing and Midwifery Code of Conduct (NMC 2008)

Doctors, like other professionals, may feel unsure, isolated and lacking support when making decisions, and may welcome collaborative decision making. However, a study by Uden et al (1992) suggests that doctors are more likely to seek such support from superiors rather than requesting the cooperation of nurses. As one nurse said:

I have frequently felt uncomfortable about treatment decisions that are made as to whether or not to continue feeding... they [the doctors] certainly don't invite opinions from others. When I have questioned them about their decisions, I've been surprised at how unsure they are about what to do.

Rather than feeling excluded, nurses may need to promote the fact that they want to contribute. Surely it would be best in these extreme and difficult situations to work together and to value each other's contributions. The nurse may have a role as an advocate, or in providing alternative solutions. This in itself is empowering rather than frustrating and demoralising.

Whilst the results of this small study cannot be generalised, they nevertheless mirror findings in previous studies (Erlen and Frost 1991, Holly 1993). Ethics in nursing is still predominantly perceived to be restricted to the big dilemmas which, by their very nature, are, or should be, interdisciplinary. These issues invariably have no satisfactory solutions and leave those involved with feelings of frustration and dissatisfaction.

The role of ethics in everyday nursing interactions

Having listened to nurses' stories over the years, I believe that there is a much wider remit for nursing ethics, and there is evidence that this is emerging. Nursing ethics is a discipline even now in its relative infancy, and the profession is still trying to establish just what nursing ethics is (Melia 1986, Allmark 1995). Although nurses failed to articulate day-to-day nursing activities as ethical issues, nearly all nursing practice has an ethical component. Good nursing must be value based. Ethics need not be something that is only ever brought out of a cupboard when all else has failed to find a satisfactory answer. Such an approach would inevitably engender negative feelings of frustration and disempowerment in the ethical agent. Indeed, in such cases there are often no really acceptable solutions to find. Instead, nurses can use ethics proactively; examining issues in everyday practice from an ethical perspective and reflecting not only on what we do but also on what we ought to do. This process of ethical reflection should assist the practitioner to see that ethics is an essential component of all aspects of practice.

As a lecturer I have been privileged to hear nurses recount and explore values, experiences and dilemmas in practice. Perhaps these stories and others like them are the real issues for nursing ethics. The stories which follow are reproduced here with the kind permission of some practitioners. Student nurses are often well situated to identify the ethical issues in a placement area. They enter the environment without the hindrance of established practices and customs and often with a good measure of idealism and naivety which allows them to question issues that others do not see or do not allow themselves to acknowledge. The first account is a story from a student on her first placement on a busy acute medical ward.

Story one

We have been caring for an elderly lady on our team. I don't fully understand what is wrong with her, but its terminal – some kind of cancer, I think. She has developed pneumonia and her treatment has been stopped and she is just to have 'tender loving care'. Most of the time she is confused and doesn't know where she is, she has no close relatives and no one ever comes to visit her. She needs lots of nursing and I have been involved in doing her washes, mouth care and her observations. I always talk to her and explain to her when I have finished. Sometimes she doesn't seem to hear you, but when you go to leave, she clutches your hand. Even when she seems really confused, I think she is really scared. I try to stay with her as long as I can but there are so many other things to do. I think the other staff are beginning to avoid unnecessary contact with her because leaving her is so difficult and makes you feel so guilty. The trouble is this ward is so busy ...

This account is not included here as a criticism of the ward staff caring for this lady. They are, no doubt, under great pressure with many competing interests for their time. Rather, it is included as a reminder to constantly review those fundamental values underpinning practice, and as a reminder of the need to reflect closely on what we actually do rather than what we think we do in the light of those values. Ethical reflection in nursing enables the agent to identify what ought to be, and offers an opportunity to change practice in response to that reflection. Does this care really fulfil the unique role of the nurse (as identified by Henderson 1966) to assist the patient to a peaceful and dignified death? Most of us would agree that it does not. In spite of the competing pressures, this lady should take priority over most other activities in the ward. She should have a nurse to sit with her, to support her and to assist her to a peaceful death. The justification, if one is needed, is both contextual and rational. Contextually, the patient is very clearly frightened and distressed, and it seems to be the right thing to do. More objectively and rationally, duty-based and consequence-based theories both agree that individuals are fundamentally equal. Therefore we should be able to make an equal claim for care. Humans, simply because they are humans, are entitled to respect. If we are to be respected, our autonomous decisions ought to be listened to and, whenever possible, acted upon. Autonomy, where it does not infringe another's autonomy, ought to be respected (Beauchamp and Childress 1994). In this case, the patient has clearly communicated her wishes to the nurses caring for her. There are, however, competing interests: obviously, time spent with this lady means that time cannot be spent with other patients. Other relevant important principles to bear in mind here are those of promoting good and doing no harm. The ethical decision is, therefore, who should receive priority? Ethical reflection may take the following form: whose interests should take priority and why? It could be argued that, with the exception of life-saving measures, the needs of the other patients could wait. Communicating this to those patients may be an important aspect of this issue. The dying lady's wishes have been clearly communicated and should take priority over other, less urgent wishes. This lady is dying relatively imminently; she will only die once; there is no room to get it right next time. The harm and distress that results from not being supported at this time is very real and cannot be rectified later. Washes, drinks, and even more complex nursing activities can be delayed. There is still a pervasive belief in nursing that getting the work done is the most important nursing action. Whilst this is undeniably important, the cost of achieving that goal should not be too high. If the ethical reflector combined the above reasoning with the knowledge that avoidance tactics are probably being used to protect the nurses from the discomfort engendered by delivering inadequate care, the agent would be obliged to review how this patient's care is being managed.

Ethical reflection requires that the nurse reviews the potential consequences of particular behaviours alongside fundamental values, whilst taking into account the particular context of the issue, in order to find a right way of acting.

Story two

> *We have lots of confused and demented patients on our ward. It seems that whatever you try to do for the best turns out wrong. These patients are frequently disruptive and interfere with other patients. It's not their fault; they don't know where they are half the time. The only thing that seems to work is if you sit with them. Obviously this has an effect on the other patients; just because they are sitting quietly doesn't mean they don't need any care. So what normally happens in the end is that the noisy and disruptive patients end up being mildly sedated so that they don't get so distressed. This doesn't really solve the problem, it just hides it.*

This is the voice of a frustrated and disillusioned nurse who feels that current strategies are inadequate but who is unable to offer any alternatives. The frustrations of feeling that one is not doing the job well and that the solutions one is using are not doing good and may even be perceived as harmful, may strike a chord with many practitioners. There are, of course, no quick-fix solutions. This nurse has already taken the first steps towards improving practice. She has begun the process of ethical reflection. She has identified that this practice does not accord with her underlying values, and she has expressed the sense of discomfort that so often alerts us that this is an ethical issue. The next step is to begin to explore what the practice ought to be, taking into account the context and universal ethical principles. Reflecting on different options for achieving best practice might be the next step. This stage would preferably be done by the whole caring team, as it is likely to produce more diversity of ideas. It is important that any modifications in care management are agreed and accepted and consequently implemented by all those involved if change is to occur. Implementing and evaluating the most promising options enables the practitioner to regain a sense of empowerment and a control of their practice as well as potentially improving the patient's experience.

Story three

I work in a busy rehabilitation unit.The patients who we treat have usually suffered some catastrophic event which has changed their current and future lives. Patients are referred to us because they are likely to make significant progress and benefit from intensive rehabilitation.The staff in the unit are all committed to rehabilitation and promote a very positive attitude to the patients. Before they arrive with us, a rehabilitation programme is worked out with the multi-disciplinary team. We try to integrate the patients into the ward very early and encourage them to use the communal spaces when they are not booked for rehab sessions. There is a fairly strict routine in the ward: the patients get up early so that they are ready for the physiotherapy and occupational therapy sessions at 9 o 'clock; lunch is served in the day room at 12.30 and then there is a rest hour following lunch and prior to more rehabilitation sessions. The patients are usually tired at 10 o'clock and the night staff try to get the ward lights out early.

I was very proud of the positive environment that we convey in our ward until this was questioned by a patient who had been sent by their consultant to rehabilitate. No one had asked what they hoped to get out of the experience or indeed if they wanted to rehabilitate. They objected to getting up early in case the porter came to take them to the gym for their session. They had not eaten communally for some years and did not intend to start now. This caused me to stop and think about what we were doing, and for whom? Since that time the ward has begun to change; patients are much more closely involved in discussing what they hope to achieve and why they think they are with us. Appointment times are now made for all patients attending physiotherapy and occupational therapy, and are tailored to suit individual preferences where possible. Patients are asked where they would like to eat.

These are only small changes and have interestingly met with some resistance from staff members, but this is only the beginning ...

This story needs little comment. It is a good example of a practitioner who reflected on existing practice and who, whilst thinking it had been good, was prepared to review it. In fact, it resulted in her reviewing her own personal and professional values, and subsequently challenging the values of many of the team members. The result was an attempt to improve practice in the light of these reviewed values, the most prevalent of which has been the promotion and respect of patient autonomy. Listening to what the patients actually want, rather than what it is perceived that they want, has been a significant change in this unit.

It is easy to forget how powerful both the institution and we, the professionals, are. The needs and wishes of the individual patient can easily be overlooked in our attempt to impose norms and particular standards of behaviour on our environment. There is an old Chinese proverb that claims: what is ethically relevant is not understanding what it feels like to be me in that person's shoes, rather it is important to understand what it feels like to be that person in that person's shoes. This may be a very tall order, but it is an ideal to which we should be able to get closer if we reflect ethically upon our practice.

The three stories above are merely an illustration of how pervasive ethics is in nursing. The really important ethical decisions in nursing are those that occur in our everyday practice; the things that really make a difference for those in our care. It is about such things that we can pose the questions: 'How and why do I do the things that I do?' and 'What should I be doing?'

Ethical reflection

Ethical reflection affords us not only with the opportunity of 'extraordinarily re-experiencing the ordinary' (Schön 1987: 93), but also provides a vehicle through which we can find ways to change and improve the ordinary. Ethics is a practical discipline, and ethical reflection is an essential tool for all practitioners.

It need not be practised in splendid isolation but can be used as a team-building and strengthening tool. Exploring and implementing shared values and beliefs about care allows practitioners to manage change and to gain a sense of personal control in their work.

Nurses should, of course, contribute to the big ethical debates in healthcare, but there may be little satisfaction from such insoluble problems. More satisfying issues for nurses to grapple with may be those raised by ethical reflection. To ensure that nurses give 'good care' which meets professional standards and public expectations it is essential to reflect on practice. The incidents of poor care that have been highlighted in Care Quality Commission Reports (CQC 2011) and the Ombudsman Report (House of Commons 2010) suggest that at least some nurses are failing to meet good standards of care. If failing to find time to do the 'little things' (Pearcey 2010) depicts practice it is necessary to reflect on what is being done and how this can be changed in order that the little things can be accommodated. These are the elements of care that make a significant difference to the recipient and distinguish good and caring nurses from average nurses. Nurses are not only accountable for the quality of the care that they personally provide, but are also held accountable for failing to act after witnessing poor care by others.

Ethical reflection requires practitioners to think critically about their values and to ensure that these values are integral to the care they provide.

Nurses must continue to ask themselves:

- What are my values and underpinning philosophy of care? (What do I believe about the nature of care and the duties I as a professional owe to those in my care?)
- How integral are these values and philosophies to the care that I provide? (Always? Sometimes? Never?)
- What compromises my ability to put my values into practice?
- How flexible is my practice in accommodating individual needs and how effectively do I work in partnership with those in my care?
- Are my decisions and actions consistent and morally justifiable? (Could I account for and be comfortable with the reasons behind my actions, if called on to do so?)
- If I am frustrated or disempowered in relation to the implementation of value-based care in my practice, what strategies do I have for changing my sense of disempowerment?
- Do I contribute effectively to the wider bioethical debate?

Work by Bergum (1994) suggests that in order to care ethically it is necessary to refocus our professional foundations:

- To move away from a position of professional dominance in the relationship with those in our care and to move towards a position of true collaboration.
- To adjust the view that only issues seen in the abstract can find the right answer and to move towards a position where the abstract is modified by the particular contextual issues.
- To change the traditional focus of care from that of beneficence, which is often paternalistic and controlling, to that of nurturance: the subtle change from 'caring for' to 'caring about'.

Ethical reflection can make a difference to patient care; it can also empower professionals to retain control of their own practice and assist them to deliver it in the manner that is consistent with their own professional values.

By reflecting on care, being more receptive to alternative ways of addressing issues, taking responsibility for the way that care is delivered and by working collaboratively with patients and colleagues, the nurse should be able to identify better ways of practising. There is unlikely to be just one right way of doing things; most decisions are a matter of judgement (Johns 1998). Professionals have choices about what they do and how they do it. Learning the language of ethics and recognising that all nursing activities have a moral component should assist nurses to deconstruct and reflect on practice and to determine ways of doing this better; it will also assist in the articulation and justification of their practice and their decisions, both to others and to themselves.

It would be wrong to leave the reader with the impression that ethical reflection is easy or comfortable; often it is not. Practitioners may well share the sentiments of a nurse in an ethics class who was bemoaning the fact that I had made her role much harder:

> *Two or three times a day, now, I find myself really questioning my practice; at times it makes me feel quite insecure.*

Ethical reflection asks the practitioner to review and modify practice in order to provide consistently good and ethically justifiable standards of care. I could be criticised for being unrealistic, but I make no apology for this idealism. It will not always be possible to provide optimum care. However, if you aim for the ideal and, due to circumstances settle for a little less, it must be better than settling for mediocrity or worse. At times ethical reflection may enhance the practitioner's feeling of disempowerment. This is often true when it is not possible to resolve issues being tackled to everyone's satisfaction. There will always be some things that we are unable to influence. If we have identified that this is indeed the case and that there are no creative solutions, we may need to let go until such time as the conditions have changed. Ethical reflection does not require practitioners to hit their heads against a brick wall. Knowing and accepting that some things are out of our control is an important lesson for us all to learn. Indeed, just knowing this may help us to cope with it.

I believe that ethical reflection is essential for the provision of good care. Caring is a moral activity. It must involve the application of values. In a service in which standards are articulated, regulated and inspected, individual practitioner behaviour is crucial. Delivering and measuring quality care is not the same as measuring quality control in a factory producing inanimate goods. There is no universal package of care delivery that applies to all people. Each patient requires something individual and unique. It is the responsibility of the professional to reflect on what that person needs and to ensure that standards of care are met, that best evidence is used and that competent practice is adhered to. However, in addition, ethical reflection requires that more than this occurs. Ethical reflection requires that the professional reflects on the attitude and manner in which that care is provided.

Ethical reflection provides a platform from which professionals can gain a deeper understanding of their practice. I suggest that it improves care because it asks practitioners to not only provide competent care but also to understand and defend the manner in which care is given. Practice that is based on ethical reflection has much more chance of meeting public and professional expectations than that which is not ethically founded. Ethical reflection empowers the practitioner as it enables practitioners to articulate a moral account of their practice.

Points for reflection

The following issues have been raised within this chapter:

- In order to care ethically it is necessary to reflect on both personal and professional values.
- Care practice is a moral activity and values are as integral to good care delivery as is knowledge and skills.
- Ethical reflection provides practitioners with a deeper understanding of the

manner in which they practice and provides a framework for change.

- Ethical reflection can empower the care practitioner.
- Ethical reflection requires that practitioners take responsibility for the standards of care that they provide and requires that they reflect on the care that they see others provide and act on this where appropriate.

References

Allmark P (1995) Uncertainties in the teaching of ethics to students of nursing. *Journal of Advanced Nursing* **22**: 374–8

Beauchamp T, Childress J (1994) *Principles of biomedical ethics.* Oxford University Press, New York

Benner P (1984) *From novice to expert: Excellence and power in clinical nursing practice.* Addison-Wesley, California

Bergum V (1994) Knowledge for ethical care. *Nursing Ethics* **1**(2): 71–9

Care Quality Commission (2011) *Dignity and nutrition inspection programme. National Overview*. Newcastle, Care Quality Commission

De Wolf M (1989) Ethical decision making. *Seminars in Oncology Nursing* **5**: 77–81

Erlen J, Frost B (1991) Nurses' perceptions of powerlessness in influencing ethical decisions. *Western Journal of Nursing Research* **13**(3): 397–407

Department of Health (2003) *The essence of care benchmarks*. Department of Health, London

Gaul A (1987) The effect of a course in nursing ethics on the relationship between ethical choice and action in baccalaureate nursing students. *Journal of Nurse Education* **26**(3): 113–7

Gilligan C (1982) *In a different voice: Psychological theory and women's development.* Harvard University Press, Cambridge

Glaser B, Strauss A (1967) *The discovery of grounded theory: Strategies for qualitative research.* Aldine Publishing Company, New York

Grosenick L (1994) Government ethics and organisational culture In TL Cooper (ed) *Handbook of administrative ethics* (pp 183–197). Marcel Dekker, New York

Health and Social Care Act (2008)(Regulated activities)Regulations 2010 (SI2010/78)

Henderson V (1966) *The nature of nursing: A definition and its implications for nursing practice, research and education.* Macmillan, New York

Holly C (1993) The ethical quandaries of acute care nursing practice. *Journal of Professional Nursing* **9**(2): 110–5

House of Commons (2011) *Ombudsman report into the care of elderly people.* House of Commons, London

Husted G, Husted J (1991) *Ethical decision making in nursing.* Mosby, St Louis

Johns C (1998) Unravelling the ethics of a good decision. *Nursing in Critical Care* **3**(6): 281–2

Ketefian S (1989) Profession and bureaucratic role conceptions and moral behaviour among nurses. *Nursing Research* **34**: 248–53

Kuhse H, Singer P, Rickard M (1993))artial and impartial ethical reasoning in health care professionals. *Journal of Medical Ethics* **23**: 226–32

Leininger M (1988) *Caring: An essential human need.* Wayne State University Press, Detroit

Lipsky M (2010) *Street-level bureaucracy: Dilemmas of the individual in public services.* Russell Sage Foundation, New York

Melia K (1986) The task of nursing ethics. *Journal of Medical Ethics* **20**: 7–11

Milton Wildey K, O'Brien L (2007) Nursing care of older patients in hospital: Implications for clinical leadership. *Australian Journal of Advanced Nursing* **28**(2): 6–16

Nursing and Midwifery Council (2008) *The code: Standards of conduct, performance and ethics for nurses and midwives.* Nursing and Midwifery Council, London

Pearcey P (2010) Caring? It's the little things we are not supposed to do anymore. *International Journal of Nursing Practice* **16**: 51–6

Peter E, McFarlane A, O'Brien-Pallas L (2004) Analysis of the moral habituality of the nursing work environment. *Journal of Advanced Nursing* **47**: 356–67

Schön DA (1987) *Educating the reflective practitioner.* Jossey Bass, London

Seedhouse D (1998) *Ethics the heart of health care* (2nd edn) Wiley, Chichester

Tronto J (2001) An ethic of care. In Holstein M, Mitzen P (eds) *Ethics in community-based elder care.* New York, Springer Publishing

Uden G, Norberg A, Lindseth M (1992) Ethical reasoning in nurses' and physicians' stories about care episodes. *Journal of Advanced Nursing* **17**: 1028–34

Yarling J, McElmurray E (1985) The moral foundation of nursing. *Advances in Nursing Science* **8**(2): 63–73

Suggested further reading

Health Ombudsmans Report (2010) *Care and Compassion? Report of the Health Ombudsman on ten investigations into NHS care of older people.* Stationary Office, London

Nursing Ethics: An international journal for healthcare professionals. Amold Hodder Headline, London

Chapter 3

Taking it on the chin

Paul Ward

RMN training

Final placement: acute psychiatric admission ward

Third shift: early: I was punched in the face by a patient today!

A new admission had come in over night. A 32-year-old woman with a history of manic-depression who was currently hyper-manic had been a compulsory admission under the then Mental Health Act and this was the main source of her anger. The woman was extremely active, wandering the ward and regularly trying to leave. Her mode of speech was causing some problems, as she talked fast and furiously to anyone who would listen. In fact, it did not matter whether anyone was actually listening or not, she would shout at them anyway. She would shout about the injustice of being 'imprisoned' there against her will and would shout at the nurses, using as many expletives as possible. She would be personally insulting and seemed to be particularly adept at targeting personal characteristics about which the individuals singled out were obviously sensitive. This was causing problems with other patients whose reactions were varied, depending on their current problems. For some the woman's behaviour fed into their paranoia; for others she was the devil come to torment them. One patient sat quietly brooding. He was always a powder keg waiting to blow and the general feeling was that this woman was likely to be the match to light the fuse. Other, more sensitive souls, would scuttle away, sobbing – everything felt uneasy and unpredictable.

The situation was also causing problems for the caring team. The night staff were looking particularly jaded. They had been on the go since midnight and their patience was wearing thin. The sight of the day staff drifting in was obviously a blessed relief.

As a student nurse it seemed to go with the territory that I got all the jobs the permanent staff disliked. I found it difficult to address this and to enter any meaningful discussion on the subject. 'We have all had to cope with crap as students. How else are you going to learn?', was the usual reply from other nurses. I was therefore assigned to 'closely observe' the woman. This is also known as 'one-to-one', 'level one' or 'level three' care, depending on where you work. It involves virtually shadowing the person, ensuring that they stay on the ward and that they come to no harm either from their own or others' actions. In theory this seems fairly straightforward – perhaps the only alternative to locked wards. In practice it is a complete nightmare, both for the observer and for the observed. It ensures that the nurse ends the shift feeling both drained and dehumanised from constant abuse. It is certain that the patient feels the same, but he or she cannot go home at the end of the session. Instead there is another fresh face to contend with. The procedure also appears to serve the function of making the patient's symptoms worse: increasing frustration, paranoia, and anger and then leading inevitably to aggression and violence directed towards the perceived oppressors.

This was my fate for the day, and my worst fears were realised. The more I followed the woman, the more she tried to lose me. The more I tried to communicate with her, the more she twisted my words and abused me. I felt inexperienced, and ill-equipped to deal with the situation. The other members of staff found my discomfort and embarrassment a great source of amusement. It was plainly obvious that the woman was finding the situation of a six feet four male following her around and watching her every move very threatening, as anyone would. Every effort on my part to communicate this perception to the qualified staff nurses seemed to fall on deaf ears. I felt that they were thinking I was trying to get out of the job – a job that was plainly the most difficult that day and needed an experienced approach to avoid a disaster occurring.

I was constantly assured that this was what mental health nursing was all about and that I would soon get used to it – this was the only way to learn. Perhaps this was true, but surely some guidance might be useful. As usual, my mentor was on a different shift and everyone said, 'Talk to her when you see her'. All well and good, but I needed help there and then. It all came to a head when, after one particularly long tirade, the woman bolted up the ward towards the main door. I was in pursuit, trying to maintain any remaining shred of dignity that I thought either of us might have. As I rounded the corner, I came up against what felt like a brick wall but what was, in fact, a well-aimed fist to my jaw. I reeled back, mostly in surprise, tripped against a chair and fell flat on my back. Before I was able to gather my senses, male staff were everywhere. The woman was restrained using holds which, I am sure, have never appeared in any recognised control and restraint manual, and then marched to her room. The ward had suddenly become alive; other patients were ushered into the day room, keys jangled, syringes were drawn up and doors banged, whilst I nursed the mother of all headaches. Where had all these people been when I had needed them earlier? Nothing happened after that, except that I became the butt of the joke for the rest of the shift and I was asked to fill in a form about what had happened. That was it. The incident was soon forgotten. Not by myself, however. I had no physical scars but I was left feeling angry, humiliated and let down by my colleagues.

We, as mental health professionals, are generally perceived as all-powerful in the eyes of the patient (Johnson et al 1997). This is by dint of our 'legitimate power' because our actions are sanctioned by society, and our 'expert power' because we are seen to have insight and skill (Price and Mullarkey 1996). Generally, this professional power is accepted by most people under our care because they know they ultimately hold the trump card – they can refuse treatment and discharge themselves if necessary. This, however, was not so for my Sectioned patient; she could not leave or refuse treatment; I was her gaoler and tormentor, acting on behalf of an oppressive regime. The balance of power was tilted in my favour, yet why did I feel so disempowered? Maybe Price and Mullarkey (1996: 17) have the answer:

> *... paradoxically, the client potentially holds the most powerful factor in the relationship: namely resistance, in particular to an authority figure – the nurse.*

Certainly she resisted in the only way she knew how – by hitting back. It felt that this was her 'right' and there was nothing I could do about it. Maybe she knew that she could get away with it because, after all, that is what mentally ill people do, is it not? This seems to be the popular perception, that surely we cannot expect to work with the mentally ill and not get hit now and then? We must accept it, it's all part of the job, an occupational hazard. Is this really how it is? Something that has always happened and will always happen? Is it something that we cannot change. Psychiatric patients will be aggressive and violent, and mental health nurses the natural targets?

The important issue here seems to be that nurses feel disempowered when faced with aggressive and violent situations, and that perhaps the only way they can feel empowered in relation to this is to respond to like with like; they are human after all (Chambers 1998). This response is perhaps legitimised by official control and restraint training. How can nurses empower themselves and move away from the 'accept it and respond when necessary' approach that appears to be the culture? I have a vested interest here to find an answer to this question because I do not want to continue with my chosen career as a sitting target, however inevitable the cultural norm expects that to be.

How should it be? I believe that we, as mental health nurses, should be exploring ways of preventing aggression and violence on the ward, thus empowering ourselves with prevention over cure and, in turn, inevitably empowering our clients so they do not have to use aggression and violence as a means of communication. In this way we would achieve a more even balance of power. Am I being naive here? Will I, in a few years time, come to realise that this is simply how it is for mental nurses and patients? Perhaps the stereotypical view that all psychiatric patients are violent goes much deeper than I realise, and manifests from a much wider social perspective. Certainly it is a view perpetuated by the media which influences the popular view, that anyone who works with psychiatric patients must surely expect to be assaulted at some point or another (Waterhouse 1994). Mental health nurses and patients are, perhaps, as much influenced by the media as is anyone else.

There is a general perception that aggression and violence are problems which are increasing in society generally, and that it is understandable to expect such a trend to be mirrored in healthcare settings. Not only the output of the media, but also anecdotal evidence from the mental healthcare profession itself, continues to feed the expectation that aggression and violence is an occupational hazard. Breakwell (1989) acknowledges that values held by many in the caring professions show an acceptance of a certain level of 'tolerable aggression' from those in their care. She expresses the view, however, that these values may now be shifting towards zero tolerance, which I find encouraging in my current frame of mind.

When I performed an initial search through the academic literature on the subject, I was presented with many titles. Most have recent dates and, at face value, seem to echo Breakwell's sentiments and highlight that I am not alone in being assaulted. The catalyst for the flurry of writing on the subject appears to have been a national survey conducted by the Health Services Advisory Committee (1987). Up until this point it seems that most research tended to be small, locality-specific and often anecdotal, making it difficult to generalise across the overall population of healthcare settings. Whilst the 1987 survey seems to have its own limitations, it certainly did much to highlight the experience of healthcare staff and to bring the subject onto the professional agenda. There is much evidence to suggest that nursing is a high-risk occupation for assault (Whittington 1997, Stephen 1998, Vanderslott 1998) and the indications seem to be that the highest incidence of assaults to staff occur in psychiatric settings. Whittington (1997) reports that the number of assaults against nurses are skewed in these settings and quotes averages of one assault in every 11 days. Perhaps there is some truth in the stereotype?

Back in 1991, the National Union of Public Employees (NUPE) published a survey which found that 87 per cent of nurses interviewed were worried about violence. NUPE maintains that official statistics 'grossly underestimate' the level of violent threats made against nurses, with almost nine out of 10 questioned saying that they had felt threatened at some time. All of these showed signs of distress lasting many weeks after the event (NUPE 1991). It is also significant that Collins (1994) found a high rate of agreement with the statement:

> *Staff working with mentally ill people can expect to be physically assaulted some time during their career.*

Interestingly, one explanation given for this was that because there is so much literature suggesting that nurses can reasonably expect to be assaulted, it then becomes a self-fulfilling prophecy (Collins 1994).

Some of the literature appears to support my own reactions to patient assault. Lanza et al (1991) reported reactions that included emotional, cognitive, social and biophysical responses, often lasting up to a year, well beyond the return to work. It was also found that staff often had to ignore or minimise their reactions in order to continue. This may explain the other nurses' reaction to my assault as it perhaps reminded them of their own experiences. It may also explain why I was the butt of their jokes and expected to join in. To laugh off and joke about assault is perhaps an understandable response when the culture persists with the perspective that this is part of the job description.

An interesting view offered by Lanoff-Bollman and Frieze (cited in Murray and Snyder, 1991) perhaps helps to explain this. They say that most people hold three basic assumptions which enable them to go about their lives and work in relative comfort:

- A belief in personal invulnerability.
- A perception that the world is meaningful and predictable.
- A view of ourselves in a positive light.

These assumptions give a sense of safety, stability and self-esteem due to the perception that the world is an orderly place. The intense feelings that staff may experience when assaulted may be due to the breaking down of these assumptions. The person's world suddenly feels unsafe and unpredictable, there is a heightened sense of vulnerability, a feeling of being responsible for the incident and a negative self-image (for example, 'I am weak and foolish').

This backs up both Lanza et al's (1991) findings and my own experience that such incidents may be minimised, joked about, and any uncomfortable feelings laughed off as trivial by other staff. I would also agree with the view that the assaulted nurse can feel to blame for the incident and somehow be seen to have done something wrong. Such mechanisms serve to maintain a perception of control for those involved, whilst avoiding succumbing to their true feelings.

It is strange that we react in this way when there is no doubt that we all experience some form of negative reaction to violence and aggression. Poster and Ryan (1993) found that anger was the most reported emotional response immediately after an assault. Then, in the weeks following, other responses reported included anxiety, helplessness, irritability, sadness, feeling sorry for the patient, and feelings that the assaulted nurse could have done more to prevent the incident. This last was my own main feeling; surely there was more we could have done to prevent this happening.

It is encouraging that the literature highlights the effects which assault has on practitioners, but it makes depressing reading. There is a certain inevitability to it all that underlines one staff nurse's comment to me: 'You can't expect to become a psychiatric nurse and not get hit sometimes.' My answer to that is: Why the hell should it? Why should we continue not only to feel powerless regarding patient violence and aggression, but also to sit back and just wait for it to happen? And why, when it does happen, can we react only in a knee-jerk fashion, using chemical or physical means to overpower the aggressor? Certainly, in this way we completely disempower our clients and ultimately perpetuate our own powerlessness. An endless cycle of disempowerment, each incident feeding the next.

If we could do as much as is possible to prevent violence occurring, surely this would go some way to breaking the cycle. But how preventable is violence? I cannot be the first to have asked these questions, so maybe I am naive in thinking that it is possible. Thomas (1995), for example, has pointed out that no one has devised a satisfactory test to predict aggressive and violent behaviour and Allen (1997) concluded that risk assessment is an inexact science.

Logic rules out the notion that demographic variables, such as age, sex, race, education and socioeconomic status, would enable the prediction of in-patient violence. Lanza et al (1996) concluded that sociodemographic factors were, indeed, unreliable as predictors and tend to be similar for the population in general.

I have noticed that psychiatric diagnosis is sometimes said to be a useful predictor, but this could present problems. Many patients can have more than one diagnosis, making it difficult to isolate the different effects. Also, it is apparent that two people with the same diagnosis do not necessarily behave in a similar way. Indeed, Davis (1991: 590) concludes that

> *... patients with the same diagnosis may manifest different behaviour at different times, making diagnosis an unreliable predictor of incidents.*

Despite this, a number of the staff nurses on our ward felt diagnosis to be a good predictor. One believed that: 'If you can stabilise the illness, then you stabilise the violence and aggression.' Another stated, 'You can pick out someone who's going to be aggressive by the type of illness that person has got.' The majority of staff, however, tended not to use diagnosis as a predictor alone but many did place significant emphasis on it. Whilst such diagnosis may be useful to 'put you on guard', it does continue to fuel the stereotype of violence in certain illnesses, such as schizophrenia.

Generally, stage of illness rather than diagnosis alone is a more useful predictor. Patients with psychotic disorders, for example, have greater potential for violence in the acute phase of their illness (Stuart and Sundeen 1995). Sheriden et al (1990) noted that drugs and alcohol misuse play an important part in violent behaviour. Their findings suggest that substance misuse occurs more often in patients than is generally identified on admission. This is significant because I have since discovered that my assailant had in fact been misusing amphetamines for some time prior to her admission.

Sheriden et al (1990) and Blair (1991) view history of violence to be the most common factor associated with violence on admission. Palmstierna et al (1991) also found that people with a previous history of violence and drug misuse were significantly more likely to behave violently as in-patients. The authors conclude, however, that these findings have limited value for reliable prediction.

Davis (1991) reports on studies which highlight a variety of behavioural cues, which in turn correlate with violent behaviour. These include tension, mannerisms, posturing, suspiciousness and uncooperativeness. Whittington and Patterson (1996) found easily identifiable signs of imminent aggression, such as verbal abuse, abnormal activity and threatening posturing. Awareness of verbal and non-verbal behaviours such as these should allow the nurse to predict imminent assault and perhaps to take preventative action such as the employment of de-escalation techniques (Stevenson 1991).

Psychiatric patients are likely to have low self-esteem and this can be exacerbated significantly by compulsory admission and enforced compliance with medication. As I have already observed, violence is, perhaps, the only way these patients feel they can achieve their desired needs.

Situational and environmental factors are believed to play a role in violent behaviour, and these include aspects of setting and the presence of staff and other patients. A number of writers have recognised that violence is interactive in that aspects of the in-patient's environment can affect that person's behaviour. Lanza et al (1994) maintain that situational factors are a key variable in the prediction of violence. They also cite other research which concludes that environmental factors have more significance than diagnosis in predicting violence.

A common occurrence in the studies is that violence is in some way provoked by environmental factors and is not simply the result of some underlying pathology. It is important to remember this. Many of these factors are significant in relation to my own incident. Certain studies, for example, found that the number of incidents varied according to the time of day (Lanza et al 1997). Eighty per cent of all incidents in Convey's study (1986) occurred between 8.00am and 8.00pm, and over one third were directly influenced by mealtimes. Lanza et al's (1994) findings show that most assaults occurred in the ward corridors. Lanza et al also suggest that situations such as overcrowding and lack of space and privacy are important issues. Maybe it is noteworthy that my incident occurred in a corridor at around breakfast time. There is a significant amount of research to reflect upon in the field of aggressive incidents (Pearson et al 1986, Paxton et al 1997).

It is significant that many writers point to the environment as affecting the incidence of violence (Johnson et al 1997). Our unit has narrow corridors with low ceilings and no natural light. The TV constantly blares out of the dayroom and smoke and music billow out of the smoking room next door – hardly conducive to relaxation and 'getting your head together'. Stevenson (1991) supports the view that a calm, quiet environment is essential in order to reduce anxiety and anger in patients experiencing frustration. Too quiet and calm, however, would surely induce boredom which is itself another factor influential in precipitating aggression (Stuart and Sundeen 1995).

A report by Davies (1994) which investigated the conditions of a similar unit to the one where I work, indicates that one of the worst problems was that nurses could not see the patients due to the design and layout of the building. The layout of our unit, with its blind corners, has caused considerable problems, not least for myself, with a fist waiting for me as I rounded one of them.

More importantly for me, there has been significant interest in the issue of provocation. Blair (1991) maintains that provocation is an important risk predictor because the issues can be recognised, assessed and then appropriate interventions can be implemented to reduce the associated risks. He points to involuntary admission, physical or verbal limit-setting and staff attitudes as factors which can provoke a violent incident.

All of these factors are significant in relation to my incident. Certainly the fact that the woman had been admitted to our ward under the Mental Health Act was a key factor in initiating her violent response. This, together with limit setting in terms of preventing her from leaving the ward, added to the strength of her reaction. One staff nurse told me after the incident that, 'People who want to go out and are on a Section usually get aggressive.' Why was I not told this before? Going on this insight alone, my incident could have been predicted and thus prevented from reaching the stage which it did.

The use and effect of close observation appears a great deal in the literature, and most authors consider it to be a factor which provokes aggressive reactions. The ward policy states that if patients are believed to be a danger to themselves or to others, then they must be closely observed. Lowe (1992) cites the merits of monitoring the patient, yet most experienced staff believe that this often provokes aggressive and violent outbursts. The same staff nurse told me, 'Close observation causes or creates aggressive behaviour; people should always be aware of that.' This underlines the fact that I should not have been closely observing the patient; a staff member more skilled and experienced should have been given the task. Vanderslott (1998) cites studies which show student nurses to be the most likely grade of staff to be assaulted. Inexperience and poorly developed patient relationships due to short-term placements were put forward as likely explanations. Moreover, Lowe (1992) concludes that staff who are skilled in close observation will be able to recognise behaviour patterns, where ability places them in a very good position to prevent these patterns from escalating into violent action.

Morrison (1993) and Sheriden et al (1990) suggest that many violent patients view their staff victim as having provoked the attack. Davis (1991) points out that these patients claimed both provocation by staff and teasing by other patients as triggers for their violent behaviour. I am certainly aware that my following the female patient around may have provoked her attack on me. Ray and Subich (1998) suggest that staff attitudes can provoke aggression and violent behaviour. When staff act in an authoritarian, rigid or intolerant manner, patients may then try to regain control by using violent behaviour. Whittington and Wykes (1996) found that frustrating patients by limit setting, and intruding into their personal space stimulated them to respond violently.

Finally, Davis (1991) speculates that in-patient violence can be created by what he calls a 'norm of violence' on wards; there is an expectation that aggression and violence is acceptable and will be tolerated. This expectation may have evolved through an inflexible, non-therapeutic milieu which can make it difficult for staff to respond empathetically. The patients, in turn, see the ward as threatening and coercive, and perhaps believe that their only option is to react aggressively or violently. Such factors will create the very behaviour that staff are trying to control.

With some forethought regarding the possible effects of certain policies and procedures, many violent incidents could be avoided. And Rauter et al (1997) show that allowing practitioners to be creative within the limits of policy can reduce the perception of rigid, authoritarian staff.

Both aggressive and violent behaviour are complex concepts influenced by external and internal processes (Finnema et al 1994, Whittington and Wykes 1996). This makes accurate prediction a complicated task which is influenced by a variety of cognitive, perceptual and clinical skills (Morrison 1993). Research examining the success of mental healthcare workers in predicting violent behaviour has found that their accuracy was 'significantly better than chance' (Thomas 1995), even when demographic factors were accounted for. Poster and Ryan (1989) point out that psychiatrists have made major efforts in recent years to stress that dangerousness cannot be accurately predicted. They found it interesting that, in spite of this, their study showed a high number of respondents indicating a belief that prediction is possible. A study by Fagan-Pryor et al (1994) concurred with these findings, and the authors cite other research papers which show a majority of nurses believing that prediction is possible.

A conclusion which could possibly be drawn from all this is that aggressive and violent behaviour is precipitated by a combination of factors. A few writers (Allen 1997, Henderson and Robinson 1997, Fox 1998) have made some progress in developing risk assessment models. Significantly, these take into account multiple factors which can influence violent reactions.

So what does all this mean? Certainly I am now clear that prevention of violence is not as straightforward as I had hoped. Prediction is certainly multifaceted and can be highly speculative. However, we can go a long way in being aware of the danger signs.

The Royal College of Psychiatrists' guidelines on violence (1998) point to a number of factors which must be considered together. It is interesting that these do not seem to take into account the situational and environmental factors already discussed here, despite the importance which much of the literature places upon them. Whilst factors such as acute stage of illness, history of violence, drug and alcohol misuse, and so on, can go some way to putting staff on their guard, the guidelines still point to the 'respond if necessary' approach. All that seems to happen, for example, when an adverse risk assessment is made, is that more staff are drafted in which, in turn, serves the inevitable function of provoking a violent reaction. Around we go again!

An important point, which has become clear to me, is that we need to be more proactive when it comes to handling aggression and violence. This involves paying much closer attention to the role of situational and environmental factors in precipitating violent incidents. The literature appears to have been driving the point home for over a decade, yet it seems to have been largely ignored in the areas where I have worked.

Certainly, some environmental circumstances, such as the design of the building, are difficult to change, but as new units are built, these factors must be taken into account (Davies 1994). Other factors are possible to adjust, such as staff attitudes and how we present ourselves to the disturbed patient. Also, the practice of assigning the least experienced members of staff (that is, student nurses) to closely observe acutely ill patients should be avoided.

As mental health nurses, we must be aware of the power relationship. In the eyes of the patient, staff members are all-powerful in terms of their professional power, yet the patient potentially holds the greater power through resistance (Price and Mullarkey 1996). This is especially so where violent resistance is concerned. When faced with a violent situation, the natural human reaction is either to fight back or to run away. As mental health nurses we can do neither – our professional role will not allow it. The balance of power thus swings in the patient's favour until the nurse deems it necessary to use an officially sanctioned means of 'fighting back' , that is, control and restraint or medication. And so the struggle for power goes on until one side gives up. The patients usually capitulate, when either their symptoms become less acute or when they are medicated to the point of passive compliance, depending upon how cynical one's viewpoint is. This may seem an extreme view, and I may be bitter, but there is no doubt that this struggle for power goes on within psychiatric units up and down the country (Lipley 1998). If, by paying some attention to the many factors highlighted in the literature and discussed here, just one violent incident a week is avoided and I never get hit again, then the time and effort will have been worthwhile.

In respect of my own experience and that of the profession in general with regard to aggression and violence, I am naturally taking the route that reflects on the issue from my own perspective. I am aware, however, that there is another and probably very different perspective – that of the patient. This leads us into the contemporary issue of service user empowerment. Certainly there are pertinent questions to be asked here, such as: What are the thoughts, feelings and experiences of patients with reference to aggressive incidents? Whilst not seeking to ignore the needs of service users or to minimise their experiences, I felt it important to focus on my own needs and those of my profession in developing a more informed practice. Of course, the needs and experiences of nurses and patients are both closely interlinked as well as standing in sharp contrast.

When patients become violent they are, perhaps, responding to their own powerlessness and, at the time of violence, briefly feel empowered. That is, they are gaining some control over external factors. Empowerment is generally expressed in this way and, argues Schafer (1996), is usually difficult to achieve. He asserts, however, that empowerment expressed in terms of control over oneself is more achievable. From this point of view we, as nurses, can create the conditions for this type of empowerment to grow, rather than trying to empower our clients per se:

> *Power comes from within. You can facilitate it, but you can't make it happen.*
>
> (Wallcraft, 1994: 9)

With regard to violence and aggression, then, if we as nurses put into place the measures which help to prevent them, we create the conditions which empower our clients. Thus, we create a more positive cycle.

Initially I began this incident analysis with a view to redressing the power relationship between myself as a student and my qualified colleagues. I hoped to be able to fight my corner with the ultimate aim of avoiding being assaulted again. The analysis, however, led to my general perceptions that all mental health nurses felt disempowered when it came to patient violence, and that patient violence was accepted as an occupational hazard. It became clear to me that the only way I could hope to avoid being assaulted in the future was to look into approaches that would empower me and, hopefully, my profession. This seemed a tall order, but there are clearly numerous straightforward and well-researched measures that can be adopted. Many of these could be put into place with the minimum of fuss. Others may take more time but are still possible. I believe that, by implementing such measures, some headway can be made in redressing the balance of power, whether real or imagined, on acute psychiatric wards.

Points for reflection

The following issues have been raised within this chapter.

- There is often a struggle for power within the clinical environment and there must be an awareness of the power relationship.
- There is a need to empower newly qualified nurses to react professionally with aggressive/violent patients.

- The importance of reflection in understanding violence within the psychiatric ward, and its role in improving care needs to be recognised.
- The power relationship between students and qualified nurses needs to be redressed.

References

Allen J (1997) Assessing and managing risk of violence in the mentally disordered. *Journal of Psychiatric and Mental Health Nursing* **4**: 369–78

Blair DT (1991) Assaultative behaviour: Does provocation begin in the front office? *Journal of Psychosocial Nursing* **29**(5): 21–6

Breakwell GM (1989) *Facing physical violence.* Routledge, London

Chambers N (1998) We have to put up with it don't we? The experience of being the registered nurse on duty, managing a violent incident involving an elderly patient: A phenomenological study. *Journal of Advanced Nursing* **27**(2): 429-36

Collins J (1994) Nurses' attitudes towards aggressive behaviour, following attendance at 'The prevention and management of aggressive behaviour programme'. *Journal of Advanced Nursing* **20**: 117–31

Convey J (1986) A record of violence. *Nursing Times* **12 Nov**: 36–8

Davies F (1994) Killer building syndrome. *Guardian* **28 May**: 6–10

Davis S (1991) Violence by psychiatric inpatients: A review. *Hospital and Community Psychiatry* **42**(6): 585–90

Department of Health (1983) *Mental Health Act.* HMSO, London

Fagan-Pryor EC, Femea P, Haber LC (1994) Congruence between aggressive behaviour and type of intervention as rated by nursing personnel. *Issues in Mental Health Nursing* **152**: 187–99

Finnema El, Dassen T, Halfens R (1994) Aggression in psychiatry: A qualitative study focusing on the characterisation and perception of patient aggression by nurses working on psychiatric wards. *Journal of Advanced Nursing* **19**: 1088–95

Fox G (1998) Risk assessment: A systematic approach to violence. *Nursing Standard* **12**(32): 44–7

Health Services Advisory Committee (1987) *Violence to staff in the Health Services.* HMSO, London

Henderson S, Robinson D (1997) Developing a behavioural status index to assess patient dangerousness. *Mental Health Care* **1**(4): 130–2

lohnson B, Martin M, Guha M, et al (1997) The experience of thought-disordered individuals preceding an aggressive incident. *Journal of Psychiatric and Mental Health Nursing* **4**(3): 213–20

Lanza ML, Kayne HL, Hicks C (1994) Environmental characteristics related to patient assault. *Issues in Mental Health Nursing* **15**: 319–35

Lanza ML, Kayne HL, Hicks C (1991) Nursing staff characteristics related to patient assault. *Issues in Mental Health Nursing* **12**: 235–65

Lanza ML, Kayne HL, Gulliford D, et al (1997) Staffing of inpatient units and assault by patients. *Journal of the American Psychiatric Nurses Association* **3**(2): 42–8

Lanza ML, Kayne HL, Pattison I, et al (1996) The relationship of behavioural cues to assaultive behaviour. *Clinical Nurse Research* **5**(1): 6–27

Lipley N (1998) Trusts to get targets for reducing violence. *Nursing Standard* **12**(41):8

Lowe T (1992) Characteristics of effective nursing interventions in the management of challenging behaviours. *Journal of Advanced Nursing* **17**: 1226–32

Morrison EF (1993) A comparison of perceptions of aggression and violence by mental health nurses. *International Journal of Nursing Studies* **30**(3): 261–8

Murray MG, Snyder C (1991) When staff are assaulted. *Journal of Psychosocial Nursing* **29**(7): 24–9

National Union of Public Employees (1991) *Violence in the Health Service*. NUPE, London

Palmstiema T, Huitfeldt B, Wistedt B (1991) The relationship of crowding and aggressive behaviour on a psychiatric intensive care unit. *Hospital and Community Psychiatry* **42**(12): 368–75

Paxton R, Anslow P, Milne D, et al (1997) Evaluation of a new record system for aggressive incidents in mental health services. *Journal of Mental Health* **6**(2): 149–67

Pearson M, Wilmot E, Padi M (1986) A study of violent behaviour among inpatients in a psychiatric hospital. *British Journal of Psychiatry* **149**: 232–5

Poster EC, Ryan LA (1989) Nurses' attitudes toward physical assaults by patients. *Archives of Psychiatric Nursing* **3**(6): 315–22

Poster EC, Ryan LA (1993) At risk of assault. *Nursing Times* **89**(23): 30–2

Price V, Mullarkey K (1996) Use and misuse of power in the psycho-therapeutic relationship. *Mental Health Nursing* **16**(1): 16–7

Rauter UK, de Nesnera A, Grandfield S (1997) Up in smoke? Linking patient assaults to a psychiatric hospital's smoking ban. *Journal of Psychosocial Nursing* **35**(6): 45–6

Ray CL, Subich LM (1998) Staff assaults and injuries in a psychiatric hospital as a function of three attitudinal variables. *Issues in Mental Health Nursing* **19**(3): 277–89

Royal College of Psychiatrists (1998) *Management of imminent violence*. RCP, London

Schafer T (1996) Empowering service users: The myth, the reality and the hope. *Journal of Psychiatric Mental Health Nursing* **3**: 391–4

Sheriden M, Henrion R, Robinson L, et al (1990) Precipitants of violence in a psychiatric inpatient setting. *Hospital and Community Psychiatry* **41**(7): 776–80

Stephen H (1998) Horrifying catalogue of attacks on nurses. *Nursing Standard* **12**(50): 9

Stevenson S (1991) Heading off violence with verbal de-escalation. J*ournal of Psychosocial Nursing* **29**(9): 6–10

Stuart GW, Sundeen SI (1995) *Principles and practice of psychiatric nursing*. Mosby,

Missouri

Thomas B (1995) Risky business. *Nursing Times* **91**(7): 52–4

Vanderslott L (1998) A study of incidents of violence towards staff by patients in an NHS Trust hospital. *Journal of Psychiatry and Mental Health Nursing* **5**(4): 291–8

Wallcraft L (1994) Empowering empowerment: Professionals and self-advocacy projects. *Mental Health Nursing* **14**(2): 6–9

Waterhouse R (1994) Why did Georgina Robinson die? *Independent* **5 Dec**: 17

Whittington R (1997) Violence to nurses: Prevalence and risk factors. *Nursing Standard* **12**(5): 49–56

Whittington R, Patterson P (1996) Verbal and non-verbal behaviour immediately prior to aggression by mentally disordered people: Enhancing the assessment of risk. *Journal of Psychiatric and Mental Health Nursing* **3**(1): 47–54

Whittington R, Wykes P (1996) Aversive stimulation by staff and violence by in-patients. *British Journal of Clinical Psychology* **35**: 11–20

Chapter 4

Ageing and empowerment: Questions and dilemmas

Ian Stewart-Hamilton

Introduction

It would be easy to present this chapter as a hymn of praise to empowerment in older people. Nobody doubts that it is in principle a 'good thing', and the rest of this chapter could consist of an uncritical eulogy to this effect. However, this would miss a fundamental point. Although empowerment per se is undoubtedly good, it must be seen against a background of extensive research on other, related topics. This places empowerment in a different light – not necessarily unflattering, but certainly one indicating the need for caution and, indeed, pessimism in use. To demonstrate this point, we will begin by considering a single case study of self-empowerment. We will then consider the general issue of empowerment in later life before searching for the root causes of this in studies of psychological and social change in older people.

Our first consideration is the case study of an individual which will be used to illuminate some of the theoretical concerns about the issue of empowerment. It is customary in cases of empowerment to cite instances of triumph overcoming adversity. There are sound reasons for doing this, but it can become a little wearying to present all cases of ageing as examples of problems waiting to be overcome. The following case presents an individual who has, to all intents and purposes, always been in tune with his ageing.

Case study: Alan

Alan is 65 years old. As he himself acknowledges, his lifestyle, although superficially different, in many ways repeats that of his father, Tom. The latter led a physically active life – a keen tennis player, he gradually cut back on participating in the sport as it became too demanding physically (although he still played a fairly gentle game into his late 70s), taking up cycling and then walking. Gardening, which he had loved throughout his life, was an activity in which he could engage right up until his final months. This last period was one during which Tom came to terms with his lot. He had arranged his will, he knew death was imminent and announced it without fear, and he finally died having made peace with all who knew him. There are worse epitaphs.

As a child, Alan attempted racket sports but, unlike his father, was 'cheerfully hopeless' at them. However, he enjoyed running and, relatively unusually for one of his generation, continued to run for exercise and enjoyment after he left school. His membership of the local athletics club was used more for the facilities and the opportunities to run than for the social concerns, and running continued as a key interest throughout his middle age. Pressure of work prevented the hobby from being taken very seriously (before retirement, Alan was a successful commercial artist) until the encroachment of early old age. At about this time, triathlon was becoming recognised as a sport (for the uninitiated, this is a race comprising a long swim, a long bike ride and then a long run with no break in between the activities). Triathlon captured Alan's imagination and he began to enter competitions. At the age of 60, his performance was sufficiently good for him to be selected for the British senior men's team at the world championships, in which he obtained a creditable middle ranking. He has since represented his country internationally on other occasions.

Alan's competitive triathlete days may be numbered, however. He has contracted a painful heel spur which makes running difficult, although he still cycles and swims at a 'serious' level of training. Faced with the question of what he will do if the injury permanently prevents him from running, Alan is phlegmatic. Yes, of course he will miss running but he realises that if the heel spur does not bar him from running, then other age-related factors eventually will. However, the purpose of running is to help to keep him fit and active, and there are other ways in which these goals can be attained. The same applies to cycling and swimming; they are, of course, enjoyable, but they are a means to an end. Indeed, the trappings of success at sport are kept modestly hidden, with trophies and so on kept tucked away in his home office and not on full view in the drawing room. For once, the cliche about not winning but taking part seems apt. Pressing him further on the issue of adjusting to changing circumstances, I asked Alan what he would do if all triathlon activities became impossible.

'Then,' he replied happily, 'I would concentrate on walking.' (His wife is a keen rambler, and Alan and she go on walking holidays.) Probing, I asked what he would do if some awful accident prevented walking?

'Then,' replied Alan, 'I would do more painting.' (As a retired commercial artist, there is a feeling of wanting to paint all the uncommercial subjects business sense had prevented.) What if he became quadriplegic? Then he would try to grip a paintbrush in his teeth. Alan elaborated on this theme. He felt that everyone is given a certain level of skill and must try to attain what he or she can at that level. Over time, abilities will gradually decrease, but it is just as great an accomplishment to meet the new standards as it was to meet earlier ones. Alan has a clearly delineated life plan in which there are well-defined and realistic goals (very akin to those of his father but, although Alan acknowledges the similarities, he denies deliberate copying). Few would dispute that he is adequately self-empowered.

Alan's case is, of course, extreme. Few of us are, or will become, international athletes. However, that is not the point of the case study. Rather, it is to portray a person who attained what was realisable for himself. There is little doubt amongst those who know him that had his highest possible accomplishment been to win an egg-and-spoon race at a village fete, then the satisfaction would have been the same. The attainment of realistic ability-appropriate goals is, therefore, a clear example of how empowerment can be attained and reinforced. However, what is left out of Alan's life story is just as revealing as what is contained within it. For example, it would be fair to state that he has a relatively small circle of friends. This is not to say that Alan is in any way an unfriendly or inhospitable person – far from it. However, his emotional nutrition has tended to come from his immediate family, his work and his running. There is nothing 'wrong' with this, but it demonstrates that many other people, for whom an active social life is far more important, would not find Alan's lifestyle empowering. Concentrating on rewarding activities, and adjusting these according to circumstances, would not be a viable solution. If one's whole life has been spent enjoying social activity, how does one compensate adequately for a loss of human company? There are, of course, methods available but here the need for skilled and sympathetic intervention becomes clearer. Indeed, extrapolating from this point, it is apparent that for a person to remain self-empowered, the less other people are needed, the better. If a person relies upon attainable goals which can be afforded and are available, then self-empowerment is possible, but relying on the presence of others cannot be so easily guaranteed.

This creates a rather bleak view of empowerment in spite of a superficially optimistic air. Empowerment may be necessary, but the degree of need is tempered by the needs of the individual. Although an easy rule of thumb is impossible, it might tentatively be suggested that empowerment is most likely to succeed when it only needs to provide little support. The more it has to provide, and the more this relies upon other people, the less likely it is to succeed.

Empowerment and ageing

The general literature concerning empowerment presents a similarly guarded view of the subject. It is undoubtedly true that it is a good and useful thing in appropriate circumstances. For example, Mok and Mui (1996) report its successful use in improving the well-being of the residents in a retirement home. It is interesting to note that the researchers also demonstrated clearly to the home's staff that the empowerment also aided themselves, and was not a threat to their professional functioning (cf Sharpe 1995). Indeed, it is difficult to find any arguments against empowerment per se in the literature. However, there are many reservations expressed about the extent of its effectiveness. Perhaps the most common is the question of who controls the empowerment – if an individual has to be shown how to be empowered by someone else, is this true empowerment, or patronage? The question may at first strike the reader as ridiculous: no one, for example, would claim that Einstein had not 'properly' attained eminence simply because as a child he had to be taught mathematics. So why should the provenance of an individual's empowerment matter? However, in certain cases, older people (and their caregivers) may feel incapable of acting without the permission or (in complex cases) the advice of professionals. In such instances, providing empowerment becomes a gift to be bestowed by an 'expert', and one which further increases the sense of control which the healthcare professional has over the older person (Brown and Furstenberg 1992).

Healthcare professionals tread a thin line. Not only must they be wary of offering empowerment, but they must also be wary of taking it away (albeit for the best of intentions). For example, Beckingham and Watt (1995) note that, in trying to help older people who have fallen ill, any attempts to restrict 'unhealthy' activities may be interpreted as disempowerment and a general restriction of freedom. This raises a further knotty problem about empowerment. We have already noted that the term will mean different things to different people. In addition, it must now be noted that a withdrawal of power may in some cases be necessary for an individual's own good. And, as with the discussion above, there is no easy solution to this problem; no simple utilitarian formula to be applied in all cases. Restricting freedom is always a dangerous step, but in some cases it is best for all concerned, even if it is not appreciated at the time. This smacks dangerously of 'Nanny knows best' or worse, but as with all healthcare, some pragmatism is always needed.

However, the caveats to be attached to empowerment do not simply end with the problems of when to offer it and the personalities of the recipients. For example, ethnic grouping is likely to shape demand characteristics and perceived areas of strength and weakness (Zimmerman et al 1992).

The list could be prolonged, but the point has surely been made – there are so many caveats that it is difficult to make blanket statements about the 'correct' form which empowerment should take. Indeed, no one in the literature on ageing seems sure about what the outcome of 'successful' empowerment should be. We may have a vague idea that people should be in charge of their own lives. In some respects, this is good news. For example, a lowering of the burden on the caring professions resulting from people taking greater care of their own welfare makes economic sense. However, by the same token, so also does voluntary euthanasia. Again, of course, being empowered does not necessarily mean being 'happy'. There are many different personality types and, for some, the concept of contentment is indeed synonymous with empowerment. Others, however, are more likely to be happy only if lacking the very empowerment which others crave. What is right for Alan may be hopelessly wrong for another individual with, for example, a more sedentary lifestyle revolving around parties and other social events. Baltes (1996) demonstrates that the optimal level of responsibility and social interaction will vary markedly both between and within individuals across the lifespan. Whilst it is fair to say that no one should be allowed to abnegate all responsibility, a wish to let some things be decided on one's behalf is a sensible one (at any age), and any attempts to empower such people 'too much' will meet with justifiable resentment and unhappiness. By the same token, as we have just seen, it may be appropriate to lessen the power of some individuals who would prefer more. It is thus true to say that each individual will have an optimal level of empowerment. What this is, can only be discovered on an individual basis: no easily applied rule can or should be inflicted. However, this does not mean that we should not be aware of the issues involved. This, in turn, begs the question: What factors create the need for empowerment and why will it differ between individuals? To answer this, we need to take a step back and consider the general questions of psychological ageing and self-image.

Defining ageing

The concept of 'ageing' is surprisingly nebulous. The first problem concerns what is meant by 'age'. Chronological age (that is, how many times the Earth has been around the Sun since one's birth) is the traditional measure, but it is only a guide to other states. For example, people aged 60 years can differ enormously from each other in terms of physical and mental state. Everyday experience shows that we consider some individuals as being 'young' or 'old' 'for their age'. Therefore, a 'typical' person of a particular age is only an approximation, with room for considerable differences between the actual members of an age group. One needs only to consider the example of Alan and compare him with a prototypical man of the same age to see the considerable range possible. Indeed, the evidence indicates that the older the age group considered, the greater the spread of variability. In other words, the older the group, the more unrepresentative the 'average' becomes (Stuart-Hamilton 1994).

A further problem which raises concerns is what is meant by the terms 'old age' or 'ageing'. In a very general sense, the meaning is clear – it is a change over time. However, in that sense, an individual growing from baby to child could be said to be 'ageing'.

At one level this is, of course, true but intuitively we feel that the term is being used inappropriately. Instead, we are more inclined to accept the term when it is reserved for describing changes which occur in later adult life. Generally, researchers and practitioners adopt a rule of thumb that 'old age' begins at a person's 60th birthday (Stuart-Hamilton 1994). There are sound pragmatic reasons for dividing the lifespan into conceptual units, but one pays a price and, in the case of ageing, it is a heavy one. The biggest mental and physical changes occur in childhood and in the final years of life. Because the former ends in adulthood and the latter in death, a contrast is established which practically guarantees that ageing is seen first and foremost in terms of decay. Empowerment is thus compromised by a mental schema which casts ageing, at best, in an unflattering light and, at worst, as a blind prejudice. The reality of ageing is that it is far more capricious and resistant to objective measurement, which creates an ironic counterpoint. This can be proven by considering the supposed 'decline' in psychological powers, such as intelligence.

Ageing and intelligence

It is certainly true that if one takes the average intelligence or memory test scores for different adult age groups, then there is a statistically significant decline in people aged 60 years and over (for example, Salthouse 1991). However, this change is not valid for everybody within an age group. Indeed, about 15 per cent of older adults will retain the level of intellectual/memory performance which they have always possessed (Stuart-Hamilton 1994). Amongst the remainder, at least part of the difference in performance between older and younger adults will not be due to ageing as such, but to peripheral factors such as the increased physical frailty of the older respondents (Salthouse 1991). For example, many older adults write less quickly because of muscular and joint problems. This will obviously be disadvantageous in paper-and-pencil intelligence tests where answers must be written down as quickly as possible. Indeed, one researcher, Storandt (1976, 1977), calculated that as much as half of the difference between younger and older adults may be due to differences in speed of writing rather than to thought per se. In other words, a large part of 'ageing decline' may be a product of how we choose to measure it. This leads us to a discussion of the cohort effect. A difference in performance between two adult age groups may be due to their age difference, but equally the two groups have been educated and brought up in radically different ways (for example, compare the first two decades of a person born in 1930 with those of someone born in 1960). Therefore, the difference could be as much a matter of upbringing as of the supposed effects of 'ageing decay'. One way round this problem is to adopt a longitudinal study in which the same people are tested both when young and when old (and hence any differences are supposedly due only to ageing, since the effects of any differences in upbringing have obviously been removed). Such studies tend to find age group differences, but they are less dramatic than when a conventional age group comparison is performed (Stuart-Hamilton 1994).

This means that empowerment is compromised by a belief that older people 'must' be getting feeble-minded, which is a fiction. There are ways of avoiding this trap. In the case of Alan and similar people, a dedication to a chosen hobby may mean that sitting back and thinking about how they are decaying is simply not an option they have thought of. Other groups may not take quite such a cavalier attitude, and see even the slightest change as a harbinger of 'senility'. It is ironic that often people may fret about such things using the very same intellectual powers that they have always had. Overall, it is certainly true that many people regard later life as a period of decline (Stuart-Hamilton 1994, 1998), leading to guidelines about how older people 'should' behave which are usually not justified by the evidence. Societal norms are nearly always disempowering, and those concerning ageing are no exception.

Social ageing

There are powerful societal norms of acceptable behaviour for each particular chronological age group (often called the 'social age'). Everybody has a set of ideas about what a typical person of a particular age group should be like. These can be based on sound principles. For example, societal pressures are against children driving, drinking or having sex because these are activities not considered appropriate for the level of maturity of children. This is implicit in the phrase 'under age', and such a concept is not under serious criticism. With older people, such social age judgements can also be sensible. For example, older people are generally discouraged from taking part in physically dangerous sports such as bungee jumping, if for no other reason than that their bones are more brittle and mend less well. Even this stricture, however, cannot be followed too rigidly. The statement that a 60-year-old man should not consider participating in triathlons might be taken at face value by many people until confronted with a case such as Alan's.

However, other rulings, even at face value, smack of little more than small town puritanism. The 'correct' behaviour of an older person can be seen in terms of a set of prescriptive activities which largely involve being sedentary (dispensing wisdom and generally not being a nuisance) and a (larger) set of prohibitions (essentially avoiding anything which 'should' be the preserve of younger adults). Again, the case study above rubbishes this point. More generally, many instances could be taken, but a particularly vivid point is made by restrictions on sexual behaviour. The idea of an active sex life for an older person is stereotypically considered disgusting by many people. Before readers begin to suppose 'perfectly true, but it doesn't apply to me', consider the following concepts:

- A: the marriage of a black man and a white woman.
- B: the marriage of a 60-year-old man and a 20-year-old woman.

It is sincerely hoped that the first statement causes no concern for readers. However, how many readers' first thoughts on reading concept B were something along the lines of 'dirty old man' or 'she must be after his money'? Alternatively, what if statement B had been describing the marriage of a 60-year-old woman and a 20-year-old man? What are the first thoughts which spring to mind? Some sound practical arguments can be produced against relationships with a large age difference (probably very different interests, the problems with raising children, a lengthy period of widowhood, and so on), but it is unlikely that these were high on the list of thoughts. Instead, there seems to be a deep-rooted antipathy against older people stepping outside the boundaries of what a particular society considers to be age-appropriate behaviour. Of course, things can change as, for example, has been shown in the case of racial and sexual discrimination. Only a few decades ago, the concept of a 'mixed marriage', as described in concept A above, would have caused outrage in most sections of the community. Today, such hostility would be considered unusual (and rightly so).

It is possible to draw out the analogy between racism and ageism further and to point out the considerable similarities between the forms of prejudice found in each case. This can be useful in highlighting the irrationality behind much of ageism and, indeed, as has been observed by many authors, a good rule of thumb is to substitute 'black' for 'old' in a statement to judge if it is prejudicial (Stuart-Hamilton 1994). However, the analogy breaks down on two important issues. Firstly, the evidence against black or other racial minority groups was often based upon spurious 'scientific' evidence, such as (supposedly) statistically significantly lower IQ scores. However, as has been seen, the evidence of lower IQ scores is, alas, true for the average older person. Again, older people are generally less physically capable and are more likely to have a debilitating physical condition. Secondly, the case for racial equality is one which, on a priori grounds, is made for all social situations. The case for age equality is rather more specific. For example, older people are not generally concerned about equal employment opportunities or educational access. A simple summary is not possible but, in essence, the case is rather more about the need for recognition as an equal voice in situations where contact is made with others. In the case study, Alan does not feel lack of status. He has proven himself in an area of endeavour which younger adults would find (literally) impossible to achieve. However, it is doubtful that, even if he had done nothing more strenuous than gardening, Alan would feel disempowered, because his strength comes from the achievement of personal goals rather than from comparisons with others or with social norms (indeed, it might be argued that he is actively defying norms, although he probably would not recognise this consciously). However, not everyone is in the fortunate position of Alan, and a feeling of lack of status has obvious implications for empowerment. If X feels less competent than Y, how can X claim to have the same dignity and right to respect as Y? However, whilst such arguments may be theoretically sound, what is the practical evidence on the status of older adults?

Self-image and ageing

Such equality of recognition is lacking, as even a cursory glance at the literature reveals. This is most evident from research on the perceived status of, and self-image in, older people. First, it can be established that negative feelings about older people are strongly held, more so even than stereotypes about gender differences (Kite et al 1993). This problem is compounded by the finding that people perceive later life as a time when things will inevitably get worse, whereas other 'low status' groups (for example, children) are viewed as having the opportunity to improve (Ryff 1991). Given such findings, it is not surprising that many older people feel a lowered self-image. A telling example of this is the avoidance of 'explicit' terms such as 'old' or 'aged' when older adults are asked to describe themselves (Ward 1984). It is also pertinent to note that self-image is lower in elderly people who believe most strongly in stereotypes (Ward 1977). In other words, if one spends younger adulthood fervently believing in the dreadful nature of 'old age', then one is doomed to become the very stereotype one despised (there is an element of poetic justice in this, but it is only likely to be savoured by those with a particular taste for schadenfreude). The problem with negative stereotypes of older people is thus twofold. Aside from the harm they cause older people, they also will ultimately harm many of those who hold them. Ageism is a unique prejudice in that it is the only one where the hater has a good chance of becoming the hated. Disempowerment can be self-inflicted.

However, it is important to note that the problem of poor self-image can be overplayed. Whilst it is right and proper that we should be concerned about ageism and its effects, it is very easy to slip into portraying older people purely as victims. This, of course, only further reinforces the negative image (albeit for the best of intentions). It also creates an atmosphere in which it is easy to imagine that the only way in which empowerment can occur is by being bestowed by a member of the caring professions and that older people, if unaided by younger adults, must inevitably be miserable and stuck in a lower caste. However, findings of lowered image can be exaggerated by the way in which studies have presented their questions. Usually, questions about the status of older people are made in a manner inviting direct comparison with younger adults, or in conjunction with a consideration of a typical older person's financial state. Neither method is likely to create a roseate glow of contentment about later life. However, if adults are asked about later life without explicit comparisons being invited, then opinions from all age groups are more positive, and even optimistic (Stuart-Hamilton 1998). Thus, the extent to which we wish to see older people as having a poor self-image, or younger adults as having negative views about older adults, may in part depend upon how we ask the question.

Personality and ageing

Empowerment fits into a rather more complex picture than might at first be imagined. It cannot be seen as a gift to be bestowed by healthcare professionals and social workers on a poor, defenceless, elderly population who would otherwise, inevitably, be crushed under a weight of oppressive societal forces, fading abilities and self-doubt. Not all will need it, and for those who do, reasons (and hence responses) may be varied. This final point is supported by the findings about the various personality types and preferred lifestyles of older people (Perlmutter and Hall 1992). The stereotype of all older adults being hostile and complaining is, of course, a myth. Some individuals will be like this, but the likelihood is that they were similarly unpleasant in their earlier life. The adult personality is reasonably unvarying through the lifespan, and it would be wrong to blame ageing for every disagreeable personality trait (for example, Perlmutter and Hall 1992; Stuart-Hamilton 1994).

Researchers from a variety of backgrounds have examined personality in late adulthood, and each has devised his or her own particular classificatory system. Arguably, common to all is a judgement of the extent to which the individual is at peace with himself or herself and the world. The greater the serenity, the more 'successful' the personality type. Amongst the best known of such measures is Erikson's (1982) concept of ego integration, which argues that the final stage of life should see an attainment of acceptance and a tying-up of 'loose ends'.

Other researchers from rather different theoretical backgrounds can be argued to have said the same thing, although this is not surprising since few would argue that a life of inner turmoil and neuroticism is a good thing. If we consider the literature concerning the lifestyles of older people, then we find that, generally, those considered to be most successful are also those most at peace. For example, in Neugarten et al's (1961, 1968) celebrated studies, four principal personality types (with subdivisions) were identified. The most desirable type was the integrated personality (subdivided into: reorganisers – as one activity became physically impossible, then another was found; focused – activities were limited to a small set of feasible and highly rewarding ones; and disengaged – the deliberate abnegation of many responsibilities). Alan is arguably a very good example of an integrated personality. He is currently focused on a small band of activities, but his future plans reveal him to be a reorganiser. There are clear indicators that he will always attempt to concentrate on some form of activity and, if triathlons become impossible, other less physically demanding pursuits will be taken up in their place. Another major Neugarten trait (although less satisfactory than the integrated type) was the armoured-defensive personality (divided into: holding on – staving off decay by maintaining a high level of activity; and constricted – dwelling on what had been lost as a result of ageing). A third group was labelled passive–dependent and characterised by a reliance on others for many needs. A fourth and final group comprised the disorganised personalities, where there was clear evidence of abnormal (and dementing?) functioning. There have been other categorisations of personality types in later life (for example, Butcher et al 1991, Neugarten 1977, Thomas 1980), but all are in general agreement that there are different responses to ageing and no single type describes everyone.

It therefore follows from this that empowerment is likely to mean very different things to different people and, indeed, that some groups of older people may resent attempts at personal empowerment. For example, it is most unlikely that Neugarten's passive–dependent personalities (Reichard et al 1962 found a similar group and called them 'rocking chair personalities') would welcome attempts to make them more responsible and in control of their own lives. This raises the question of whether healthcare professionals 'should' encourage empowerment if an individual clearly does not want it. Pushed too far, such an argument begins to sound like the reasoning for a disengagement theory, but the fact remains that not everyone wants power, so should it be thrust upon them? However, given dwindling economic resources, there is a utilitarian case in favour of making individuals help themselves as much as possible, thus liberating resources for other things (cf Lloyd 1991). It would be possible to continue this debate for several more pages without gaining further ground in either direction. Which side one supports ultimately depends upon the pragmatics of each individual situation; there is no obvious blanket statement which can cover all occasions when such a decision needs to be made. Indeed, authors writing about empowerment in older people often remark upon the importance of addressing the specific context of each problem (Perkinson 1992, Scheidt and Norris-Baker 1993). However, a point has been made, namely, that empowerment is not automatically a good thing.

Conclusions

In general, later life is characterised by a decline in intellectual and memory skills, and in perceived status. This is the primary fuel for disempowerment and is, naturally, a cause for concern. Firstly, because it acts against a priori feelings of natural equality, and, secondly, because in any case, many of the supposed age-related changes are artifacts of the experiments and measures used. In other words, seeing later life as a perfect synonym of decline is erroneous. The case study of Alan vividly illustrates that later life need not be a time of physical decline (indeed, Alan is arguably physically fitter than most younger adults) and that even if decline does strike, it need not be disempowering.

However, we need to be very careful in being too enthusiastic about empowerment. Older people may, by nature of their intellect and/or personality, be optimally served by abnegating responsibility for a greater or lesser proportion of their lives. Regarding everyone as needing an equal amount of simple 'power' is counter-productive and ultimately patronising. But how does one create the right level for an individual? This places the health professional on the horns of a dilemma: remove the right of choice from the individual to too great an extent, and the individual is not only losing self-empowerment, but also is being made to function at a level below his or her abilities. This is both inefficient and, more importantly, arguably reduces self-image. However, bestowing too much responsibility on a person may be creating an irksome load, which is stretching an individual beyond his or her means and, hence, is once again inefficient and will create a lowering of self-image because the person cannot cope. The picture is further muddied when one considers that what is a source of empowerment for one person will be a source of disempowerment for another. Thus, in our case study, the physical activities and the relatively solitary life of Alan is fed upon factors which would be anathema to a more sedentary person. Empowerment must ultimately be unique to each individual.

Points for reflection

The following issues were raised within this chapter:

- Empowerment is not automatically a good thing for the elderly client.
- Society's norms may well disempower the elderly client.
- There are a variety of forms of empowerment.
- Self-empowerment is possible for the elderly client.

References

Baltes M (1996) *The many faces of dependency in old age.* Cambridge University Press, Cambridge

Beckingham AC, Watt S (1995) Daring to grow old: Lessons in healthy ageing and empowerment. *Educational Gerontology* **21**: 479–95

Brown JS, Furstenberg AL (1992) Restoring control: Empowering older patients and their families during health crises. *Social Work in Health Care* **17**: 81–101

Butcher IN, Aldwin CM, Levenson MR, et al (1991) Personality and ageing: A study of the MMPI-2 among older men. *Psychology and Aging* **6**: 361–70

Erikson EH (1982) *The life cycle completed: A review.* Norton, New York

Kite ME, Deaux K, Miele M (1993) Stereotypes of young and old: Does age outweigh gender? *Psychology and Aging* **8**: 19–27

Lloyd P (1991) The empowerment of elderly people. *Journal of Ageing Studies* **5**: 125–35

Mok B, Mui A (1996) Empowerment in residential care for the elders: The case of an aged home in Hong Kong. *Journal of Gerontological Social Work* **27**: 23–35

Neugarten BL (1977) Personality and aging. In: Birren JE, Schaie KW (eds) *Handbook on the psychology of aging*. Reinhold, New York

Neugarten BL, Havinghurst RJ, Tobin SS (1961) The measurement of life satisfaction. *Journal of Gerontology* **16**: 134–43.

Neugarten BL, Havinghurst RJ, Tobin SS (1968) Personality and pattern of aging. In: Neugarten BL (ed) *Middle age and aging*. Chicago University Press, Chicago

Perkinson MA (1992) Maximizing personal efficacy in older adults: The empowerment of volunteers in a multipurpose senior center. *Physical and Occupational Therapy in Geriatrics* **10**: 57–72

Perlmutter M, Hall E (1992) *Adult development and aging*. John Wiley, New York

Reichard S, Livson F, Peterson PG (1962) *Aging and personality: A study of 87 older men*. Wiley, New York

Ryff CD (1991) Possible selves in adulthood and old age: A tale of shifting horizons. *Psychology and Aging* 6: 286–95

Salthouse TA (1991) *Theoretical perspectives on cognitive aging*. Lawrence Erlbaum, Hillsdale, NJ

Scheidt RJ, Norris-Baker C (1993) The environmental context of poverty among older residents of economically endangered Kansas towns. *Journal of Applied Gerontology* **12**: 335–48

Sharpe PA (1995) Older women and health services: Moving from ageism toward empowerment. *Women and Health* **22**: 9–23

Storandt M (1976) Speed and coding effects in relation to age and ability level. *Developmental Psychology* **12**: 177–8.

Storandt M (1977) Age, ability level and scoring the WAIS. *Journal of Gerontology* **32**: 175–8

Stuart-Hamilton I (1994) *The psychology of ageing. An introduction* (2nd edn) lessica Kingsley Publishers, London

Stuart-Hamilton I (1998) Women's attitudes to ageing: Some factors of relevance to educational gerontology. *Education and Ageing* **13**: 67–88

Thomas H (1980) Personality and adjustment to ageing. In: Birren lE, Sloane RB (eds) *Handbook of mental health and aging*. Prentice-Hall, New Jersey

Ward R (1977) The impact of subjective age and stigma on older persons. *Journal of Gerontology* **32**: 227–32

Ward RA (1984) *The ageing experience*. Harper & Row, Cambridge

Zimmerman MA, Israel BA, Schulz Al, et al (1992) Further explorations in empowerment theory: An empirical analysis of psychological empowerment. American *Journal of Community Psychology* **20**: 707–27

Chapter 5

Empowerment, participation and rights: Healthcare conversations with young people

Tony Ghaye

The challenge

Children and young people have been telling us their experiences of using health services, at least informally, for years. They have also been telling 'us' (that is adults) what they want services to be like. The same themes are identified time and time again (Lavis & Hewson 2011). For example, YoungMinds' response to the recent NHS Listening Exercise by the UK Government in 2011, found that children and young people have specific needs, and these must be reflected in the commissioning of services.

They consulted extensively with children and young people with mental health problems and reported that they were told, loud and clear, about the types of services this group wanted. The group's experiences and needs were very different to those of adults. In their work, YoungMinds found that children and young people wanted services in non-stigmatising settings (outside conventional mainstream health and welfare centres) with a multi-agency, multidisciplinary, one-stop shop approach, available at times that suit them (YoungMinds 2011). They also found that GP Consortia, Health and Wellbeing Boards, and local HealthWatches needed to ensure that there was real engagement with a range of stakeholders, including children and young people. The danger was that this engagement might be tokenistic. As others before them, YoungMinds reported that the aim should be, to be as comprehensive as possible and engage with hard-to-reach groups of children and young people as well as those that are the most visible and vocal. Some services do respond to what they hear and improve their services in line with the views of young people but this is not happening everywhere (Worrall-Davies 2008).

A recent article by Robinson (2010) came to a similar conclusion, and cites an Audit Commission report which states that children and young people are often 'consulted but not heard'. The central question this chapter addresses is why, in a recent project that involved 997 children and young people between the ages of 7 and 14 years, in a large multi-cultural urban area, did the group feel that some services were not taking their views and experiences seriously and acting upon them? This chapter describes a children and young people's project, that had empowerment through participation as its central ethical value. The chapter tries to explain some of the links between empowerment, participation and the rights of children and young people. These three fickle friends, empowerment, participation and rights, are an unsteady trio in several interesting ways. We value participation most when empowerment and the fulfilment of the rights of children and young people come along with it. However, as we discovered in this project, highly democratic participation does not guarantee empowerment or the fulfilment of young people's rights.

The policy context

Empowerment is a term that is used repeatedly in health policy and practice. It has been described as both a process and an outcome in this book. Participation has been high on the political agenda for some time and there are good examples of participation work being undertaken. But services are not always putting the outcomes of participation into practice. Worrall-Davies (2008) states that much of the participation work that takes place is not implemented because there is often a conflict of interest between the various stakeholders. Because of this it becomes difficult to deliver services that meet everyone's requirements. Is this an easy excuse favouring the status quo or for privileging those who have always held power? Worrall-Davies argues that competing agendas can mean that children and young people's views end up ignored. Realistically, it will rarely be possible to act on everything they say. But, arguably services need to be clear about what they are able to do, and when and why this or that is not possible. With regard to 'rights', children and young people's right to participation is laid out in the UN Convention on the Rights of the Child (UNCRC) (1989). The UNCRC is based on the premise that children and young people have the same inherent worth as adults, should be afforded respect, and are entitled to preservation of their dignity, whilst recognising the particular difficulties that children and young people face in influencing decision making. The UNCRC establishes participation as a right for all children and young people, that is not limited by age, social status, disability or other characteristics of the individual, and that is voluntary and applies to all matters concerning the child or young person.

In the Executive Summary of the National Service Framework for Children, Young People and Maternity Services (Department of Health 2004) there are two relevant 'standards':

- *Standard 3: Child, Young Person and Family-Centred Services.* Children and young people and families receive high quality services which are coordinated around their individual and family needs and take account of their views.
  So it is clear. Needs assessment requires knowing what children and young people feel and think. Service improvement is impossible without healthcare professionals listening and respond appropriately to this group.
- *Standard 4: Growing Up into Adulthood.* That all young people have access to age-appropriate services which are responsive to their specific needs as they grow into adulthood.
  If we do not have a systematic, confidential and meaningful 'system' for knowing what these needs are, how can we ever claim to deliver and manage age-appropriate services?

The NHS document, *Creating a patient-led NHS* (Department of Health 2005) was produced to support NHS organisations in moving from a service that simply delivers services to people, to a service that is totally patient led, responding to the needs and wishes of those patients. The main implication of this was to require healthcare professionals to engage positively with their local populations to discover what they want from their services. This notion of 'engagement' is problematic. It is fundamental to any notion of participation and can be linked with 'involvement' and 'empowerment.' Cartwright and Crave's (2011) definition of these terms can be seen in *Table 5.1.*

Language is important and the terminology we use is critical. The Royal College of Paediatrics and Child Health (RCPCH) in its publication, *Not just a phase: A guide to the participation of children and young people in health*

Table 5.1. Some aspects of participation

Terms	*Definitions*
Involve	To inform. To consult. 'Surely we are at the heart of care and treatment? My experiences can help service improvement'
Engage	To partner. To work directly with. 'I want staff to think about opportunities for patient and public involvement at the start of all projects'
Empower	To place authority for final decision making in the hands of the patient or the public. 'We would like to see more patients and public at senior management meetings and having a real input to future strategy' (Cartwright and Crave, 2011: 3)

services (2010), uses terms which differ from those of Cartwright and Crave (2011). These are:

- *Involvement.* This describes the inclusion of children and young people in some form of decision making process.
- *Consultation.* This is the process by which children and young people are asked for their views and opinions.
- *Participation.* This is the process by which individuals and/or groups of individuals can influence the decision making process and bring about change.

In this chapter there is a commitment to considering ways in which children and young people can influence the healthcare services which are provided for them, for example, how they can be involved in designing hospitals, developing clinics, recruiting staff, assessing performance, determining healthcare priorities and distributing resources. It goes on to say that participation is about having the opportunity to express a view, influence decision making and achieve change. Children and young people's participation therefore is the informed and willing involvement of all in this group, including the most marginalised and those of different ages and abilities, in any matter concerning their health, either directly or indirectly.

In 2007 the House of Commons Health Committee published its report, *Patient and public involvement in the NHS.* A very significant aspect of listening to and learning from patients has been this patient and public involvement (PPI) initiative. The term 'patients and the public' encompasses patients, carers, service users, individuals, groups and communities. PPI defines the way in which patients, carers and the public have a voice in decisions about how healthcare services are planned, designed, delivered and evaluated. Ideally PPI operates on two levels:

- By involving individual patients and their carers in decisions about treatment and care and empowering them to make informed decisions about their health.
- By enabling patients and the public to be involved and consulted on planning, monitoring, evaluating and developing services, proposals to change services and decisions about the way services operate.

This involvement and enablement has been achieved through Patient and Public Involvement forums, Overview and Scrutiny Committees, Patient Advice and Liaison Services (PALS) and Independent Complaints Advocacy Services

(ICAS). The House of Commons Health Committee report does admit to a lack of clarity about the scope and purpose of PPI. For example the committee asks, 'Should patient and public involvement be about more accountability, better services or health promotion?' (2007: 7), and 'What form of patient and public involvement is desirable, practical and offers good value for money?' (2007: 8).

At that time, the Department of Health in the UK believed that PPI forums failed adequately to represent their communities. First, too few people were members of forums. The average for the country was eight per forum. Moreover, those people who were members tended to be older adults, often retired and there were relatively few participants from non-white backgrounds. This meant that the views of working adults, those with young families and those from black and minority ethnic groups were poorly represented. So this PPI process did not help with articulating and acting upon children and young people experiences. In short the forums were unrepresentative and failed to attract volunteers. The formation of a PPI forum generated, for some NHS organisations, a tick box culture, which precluded wider and more inclusive community engagement.

The UK Government's listening exercise on NHS modernisation has been launched. Setting out the Government's desire to modernise the NHS with the support of patients, the public and health professionals, it was announced that engagement was to demonstrate that the Government wanted to pause, listen, reflect and improve the NHS and protect it for the future. It was to be seen as an opportunity for people to share their views and have their voices heard. But listening is one thing and very different from doing something appropriate with what you have heard.

This general theme of listening to and learning from, is replicated in many publications from the Department of Health and the Department of Children, Schools and Families for England. For example, the *You're welcome quality criteria self-assessment toolkit* (Department of Health 2006) includes quality criteria against which services can assess their progress to becoming young people friendly. The You're Welcome assessment includes four criteria relating to the participation of young people and was included in the NHS operating framework for 2009/2010. The 'Healthy lives, brighter futures' strategy for children and young people's health (Department of Health and Department for Children, Schools and Families 2009) outlines initiatives to strengthen the voice of children, young people and parents in shaping services.

The requirement for and entitlement to the participation of children and young people in service design and development is also outlined in *Every child matters* (Department for Children, Schools and Families 2008). The Department of Health guidance on world class commissioning for children and young people (Department of Health and Department for Children, Schools and Families 2009), includes 11 commissioning competencies. The third of these competencies, engagement with the public and patients, places an obligation on Children's Trusts to engage young people in the commissioning process and that this engagement should move beyond consultation to meaningful roles for young people in priority setting, monitoring and service design. It also states that commissioners should actively seek the views of young people and their families, especially vulnerable and hard to reach groups of young people. Additionally, the UK Government has asked the NHS Future Forum to continue its conversations with patients, service users and professionals to provide independent advice on four important themes:

- How to make information improve health, care and wellbeing.
- How to develop the healthcare workforce to deliver world-class healthcare.
- How to ensure the modernisation programme leads to better integration of services around people's needs.
- How to ensure the public's health remains at the heart of the NHS.

What is clear from the many policy initiatives is a desire that children and young people's interests must be at the centre of health and local authority services. The current health and local government reforms present significant opportunities in this area. The challenge is exactly how the new structures will work to improve children and young people's health. The NHS Confederation (2011) sums up the present situation thus: Children and young people should have a louder voice in influencing how services are organised and delivered, as well as a greater say over their personal health choices.

Empowerment

When considering empowerment we often assume that it is a good thing, something that is desirable. This may not always be the case, but, putting that aside, empowerment with children and young people in mind, can usefully be seen to have two aspects:

- *Inter-personal* where empowerment occurs through adult/young person interaction where knowledge, values and power circulate in interesting ways. For example, it brings into sharp focus questions such as, 'Whose knowledge is worth knowing?'.

- *Intra-personal* where empowerment is a process of personal transformation, and power is created from within the self.

Both dimensions are necessary for empowerment to take place. Health professionals and other significant adults, such as family members and teachers, have a major contribution to make to the inter-personal dimension. But they can only provide opportunities as far as the intra-personal dimension is concerned. One danger is that they will exert too much control and 'power over' children and young people, thus denying them the 'space' to draw upon their own resources. Sometimes this is to do with troublesome assumptions that some adults make about how far children and young people can indeed be:

- Experts in their own lives, with competence to communicate a unique insight into their experiences and perspectives.
- Skilful communicators, employing a huge range of languages with which to articulate their views and experience.
- Active agents, influencing and interacting with the world around them.
- Meaning makers, constructing and interpreting meaning in their lives.

It is all too easy for empowerment to become something that is 'done to' children and young people so undermining the essential nature of the process itself. In other words individuals are not engaged in the process sufficiently to become empowered.

Individual empowerment of children and young people is often referred to as psychological empowerment. This relates to a number of attributes that are needed for their personal capacity to be realised. This may include building children and young people's confidence or self-worth, boosting their self-esteem, developing their coping mechanisms, or enhancing their personal skills in order for them to make health-related choices. Individual empowerment basically means children and young people feeling and actually having a sense of control over their lives. This 'sense of control' is particularly important, and is a great challenge in participatory projects involving children and young people. A sense of control over what? Real control over what? While participation arguably is a prerequisite for any empowering strategy, participation alone does not guarantee empowerment as it can often be manipulative and passive, rather than truly engaging and empowering.

Given the interlinked issues of empowerment, participation and rights, it might be useful to consider some of the following when planning a children and young people's project. For example:

- How to be clear about the aims of the project, taking into account the 'political' landscape and resources that are available.
- How to be clear about the kind and degree of participation that is both desirable and possible for all those involved and how decision-making will (or can) be shared with children and young people throughout the life of the project.
- How far you are realistic about the extent to which change and service improvement is possible, and how this determines what you say to children and young people from the outset and especially at the end of the project.
- Who you will invite to participate and how you do this. For example, how far is your group of children and young people representative of current or potential service users? Have you included children from marginalised groups, for example, black and minority ethnic children, children with disabilities? How far is this feasible?
- Which methods of participation would best suit the aim, resources and participants? How far is it preferable to employ a variety of methods and to involve children and young people in the design methods to be used?
- What would an ethical statement, clarifying issues around consent (by children/parents), confidentiality, anonymity and disclosure, look like?
- How far would it be appropriate to develop a contract of participation? Might it include rewards for children and young people who participate? If this is a large number, how will this work and what are the resource implications?
- Which members of staff (adults) will be used and in what roles? How far do they have the necessary skills?
- What are the potential obstacles to completing the project? What (if any) contingencies are there in place?

Whatever empowerment is called, it is a complex and challenging process. The source of difficulty is that it has a normative as well as an empirical dimension. For example, normatively we can say that children and young people have been 'empowered' and this can mean that they have become better able to shape their own lives and influence those things that impact on their health. Arguably this is a worthy goal. From a more empirical perspective, 'empowerment' means acquiring a number of 'things' (qualities, skills, dispositions, etc.) that make this goal achievable. So an 'empowering' process can be when children and young people acquire key abilities (more health literacy) or psychological traits (more self-confidence). A process that involves children and young people in health service improvement can also be regarded as 'empowering' when the healthcare organisations and professionals become less domineering and more inclusive, or, indeed, when their rights are introduced or become better respected and supported. In other words, 'empowerment' can refer to two sorts of change, either making gains in the extent to which children and young people can and do shape their lives for the better, or making gains in possessing the means to do so. This ambiguity between empowerment normatively conceived as a goal and empirically conceived as a means, can be troublesome if it is ignored.

One ethical challenge that is posed by much of the recent work on empowerment is about children and young people's ability to influence (or play a part in shaping) future health services. This immediately raises two challenges. First, 'shaping' is a metaphor, and the challenge here is to work out its meaning in practice. Second, the historical meanings of 'empowerment' challenge us to consider whether, as we use the term now, it should actually mean 'having more power'. What does 'shaping one's own life' mean for children and young people? Does it simply mean making one's own decisions? Can it mean active decision-making, in contrast with passive acceptance of decisions by others (mainly adults)? It would seem perverse not to include the possession of greater power as part of its meaning. If empowerment matters to us, especially the empowerment of children and young people, then it should also matter to us that empowerment can often be frustratingly ephemeral, and we should take serious note of this. Even when children and young people do manage to be involved in projects such as the one described later in this chapter, any gains can be swept away by the vicissitudes of the 'politics' and service re-configuration processes in their own localities, or the vagaries of decision making in institutions far away. Maybe we should regard even the ephemeral gains as somewhat empowering. But we should regard children and young people as even more empowered still if these gains prevail against resistance and distortion by 'other' influences and people. If we think of power in the Weberian way as the probability that one can prevail against resistance, then I suggest that this is the kind of power that must be included within any conception of empowerment in relation to children and young people.

Participation

Alderson and Montgomery (1996) defined four levels at which children and young people can participate. These are by

- Being informed.
- Expressing a view.

- Influencing a decision.
- Being the main decider.

The first three levels are contained within the UNCRC and include any child who can, firstly, understand information, secondly, form a view and, finally, is considered to be able to form a view which can usefully inform the decision making process. These four steps provide a useful framework to think about when planning for the participation of this group in service improvement. The steps raise many issues, such as children and young people's:

- Abilities to contribute.
- Interest in their own health.
- Right to a voice in decisions about their health services.
- Right to a choice in the type of health services that are provided.
- Right to be consulted (no decision about me without me).
- Potential to influence traditional commissioner and provider patterns of service.

There are some common themes that can be derived from the literature and that are identified as being important to the success of participatory work with children and young people. For example:

- *Clarity and shared understanding*. Clarity on the purpose, objectives, parameters and possible outcomes of participation is fundamental. Lack of clarity can lead to tokenism and misunderstanding about the level of involvement children and young people may have, and make it difficult to evidence change as a result of participation activity.
- *Use of flexible and appropriate methods*. The necessity of tailoring methods to be appropriate for children and young people cannot be underestimated, taking into account factors such as their age, ethnicity, gender, individual circumstances and support needs.
- *Good relationships*. The importance of the relationship between the children and young people and significant others is an issue that comes up time and time again. Children and young people say that they need to be able to build a positive relationship with a healthcare practitioner. It is not until they feel that they can trust their practitioner that they will talk openly to them about their problems and ask for advice or information.
- *Being taken seriously*. This is a vital part of a good relationship between

> adults and children and young people. It also includes showing respect. The nature of participation is seriously damaged if children and young people feel that their views are not being taken seriously by those who managed and deliver health services. There is little point in listening to children if no account is subsequently taken of their views. And the fact that children and young people express themselves differently from adults does not justify dismissing them. Too often, token efforts are made to listen to them, but little effort is subsequently made to take on board the views they express. Even where it is not possible to act on their concerns, they are entitled to an explanation of what consideration was given to them and why their wishes cannot be implemented.

Participation is a central feature of the United Nations Convention on the Rights of the Child; it holds the whole structure together (Badham 2002). Not only is participation one of the guiding principles of the Convention, it is also one of its basic challenges. Article 12 of the Convention states that children have the right to participate in decision making processes that may be relevant in their lives and to influence decisions taken in their regard, within the family, the school or the community. The principle affirms that children are fully-fledged persons who have the right to express their views in all matters affecting them and requires that those views be heard and given due weight in accordance with the child's age and maturity. It recognises the potential of children to enrich decision making processes, to share perspectives and to participate as citizens and actors of change. The practical meaning of children's right to participation must be considered in each and every matter concerning them. As a fundamental right of the child, the right to participation stands on its own. It requires a clear commitment and effective actions to become a living reality, and therefore is much more than simply a strategy.

Rights

When I talk about rights in the context of healthcare improvement, I mean the rights of children and young people to be heard and to have their views and experiences listened to and taken into account. Respecting children and young people's views and experiences means that they are not ignored. This does not mean that their opinions should be automatically endorsed. Expressing an opinion is very different from making a wise decision. But it can imply the ability to influence decisions. Central to a philosophy of respect for the rights of children and young people is that they are listened to and taken seriously. This is a commitment to valuing them as people who are capable of expressing a view.

The right to express views freely

If children and young people are to be able to express their views, it is necessary for adults to create the opportunities for them to do so. In other words, Article 12 imposes an obligation on adults, in their capacity as parents and professionals, to ensure that children and young people are enabled and encouraged to contribute their views on all relevant matters, and to provide age-appropriate information with which to form their views. This does not, of course, imply that children should be required to give their views if they are not willing or interested in doing so. Article 12 embodies a right to express views, not a duty to do so. Respecting the rights of children and young people to be heard necessitates a preparedness to create the space to listen to their views in ways appropriate to them. This may include not only role-playing and drawing (as in the project described below) but also through music, movement, dance, story-telling, painting and photography, as well as through child-to-child and more conventional adult-to-child conversations.

The right to be heard in all matters affecting them

The right to be heard extends to all actions and decisions that affect children and young people's lives in the family, school, healthcare, local communities, and at the national political level. It is necessary to exercise care in interpreting what children and young people are saying. Where they are expressing views through visual media, adults need to allow them to provide their own interpretations of their work and not pre-judge the meaning behind their representations. Similarly, it is important to understand their interpretation of words, which may, and indeed often do, differ from adults' interpretations.

The right to respect for views in accordance with their age and maturity

The weight given to children and young people's views needs to reflect their level of understanding of the issues involved. This does not mean that their views should automatically be given less weight. Children and young people are capable of understanding and contributing thoughtful opinions on many issues affecting them. This was a major outcome of the project described below. Not only are children and young people entitled, but they also have the capacity to make a contribution to their own healthcare. Even young children can, for example, describe what they like or dislike about being in hospital or going to see their doctor and why, and can produce ideas for making their visit less frightening and distressing. They can do this provided they are given appropriate support, adequate information and allowed to express themselves in ways that are meaningful to them. We found this to be so with the 7-year-old children who participated in the project described below.

The Children and Young People's Project (2009–2010): Enhancing quality and safety

A team from Reflective Learning-International comprising an experienced nurse, a school teacher and a positive psychologist were commissioned to undertake this project by a large Primary Care Trust (PCT) in England. Its aim, which originated from within the PCT as part of the Trust's on-going quality and safety initiatives, was, 'To find an efficient and systematic way of encouraging children and young people to tell "us" about their experiences of the healthcare services and to use these experiences to drive improvement conversations within the PCT'.

In collaboration with a School Nursing Service and after two full team meetings with them to discuss both opportunities and constraints and the difference between what was desirable and what was possible, a representative sample of 997 children and young people from across a large urban area were identified. A range of child and young people-friendly methods were developed to create opportunities for the participants involved to 'show-and-tell' their most recent healthcare experiences. A central and guiding ethical principle, that was successfully sustained throughout the life of this project, was that the outcomes of it were to be both *by* and *for* children and young people. This meant shifting responsibility and power away from adult direction and control and more towards the children and young people. The project plan is shown in *Table 5.2*. This was co-constructed with senior managers from the PCT, the School Nursing Team and then assessed for practicality and appropriateness by school staff who accepted our invitation to participate in the project. Although we discussed inviting children and young people who were being 'looked after' and those who might be accessed through youth centres, it was decided that, for this project, we would only access those who were currently attending school. This was a compromise.

Table 5.2. The Children and Young People's Project plan
Phase 1: October–December 2009
1. Positive engagement with 997 children and young people in 19 schools from different areas within the city. Aim to explain project purpose and processes. Secure consent. 2. Gathering of views and experiences of children in Key Stages 2 and 3 (7–14 year-olds) about their healthcare experiences, in a child friendly manner (i.e. through the use of role-play and drawing). 3. The thematic analysis of the role-play data to be validated by participants from six schools (three primary/three secondary) and then adjustments made in the light of their comments. These to be transformed into 'experiential metrics'. 4. The results of the primary school cartoon drawing task to be fed back to two primary schools to deduce the final set of cartoon characters to be used in the ICT design challenge.
Phase 2: January–March 2010
5. Establish up to six classes, from six different schools (three primary and three secondary) for the purpose of undertaking a Creative Design Challenge. This to identify the characteristics of the tools to be developed by the group (e.g. words, colours, animation, scoring, etc.) and for the group eventually to use in various health settings in the city. 6. Co-design of tools with the children and young people (aged 7–14 years) in the six different schools. Achieve two mock-ups of a technology assisted tool (a) for 7–11 year-olds and (b) for 12–14 year-olds to be validated by different groups of children and young people later. These mock-ups to include the results of the thematic analysis in (3) above which have been validated by the children and young people and transformed into 'experiential metrics'.
Phase 3: April–December 2010
7. Validation of tools by 257 children and young people from participating schools and groups of PCT staff (e.g. school nurses, schoolteachers, teaching assistants). 8. The two finally adjusted mock-ups taken back to one primary and one secondary school group. Both mock-ups used and evaluated with use of interactive whiteboard. Action and reflective conversation to be video-taped and reflected upon with full participation of children/young people. 9. Preparation of video (of what children/young people think of the tools) and PowerPoint presentation for a workshop at the national CPHVA conference in Harrogate, Yorkshire and for presentation to senior managers within the PCT.

Phase 3: April–December 2010 (continued)
10. The two technology-assisted tools to be demonstrated to senior staff within the PCT, the School Nursing Service team and to participants in the two schools in (8) above. 11. Presentation of framed photographs of children/young people from the Secondary school in (8) above who are to be involved in the final validation process. 12. Press release by Reflective Learning-International and interviews to reporters from local newspapers by children and young people involved in (8) above.

Headteachers in a selection of secondary and primary schools across the urban area were contacted through their school nurse representative. After they explained the aim and nature of the project, each headteacher was specifically asked to consent to the following.

- Initially to have access to one (or more) classes of children/young people, in their school, whose ages are between 7 and 14 years, for up to one hour (or a double period of 70 minutes) with each class in secondary schools, and a half day with classes in primary schools.
- To be open to a conversation about further school participation in the project (see *Table 5.1*).
- For Reflective Learning-International staff to facilitate;
  - A role-playing activity with each class, where children/young people are invited to develop and present a 5-minute sketch, which conveys what they feel are important aspects of seeking and receiving healthcare.
  - A drawing activity with primary schoolchildren.
  - An ICT-based creative design challenge for secondary and primary schoolchildren.
- Project staff to keep confidential notes of the outcome/s of each activity with no child/young person or school being named or identified.

From the initial invitation and clarificatory conversations we built a representative sample of schools across the urban area as shown in *Table 5.3*.

With regard to the nature of participation, we began to make distinctions between 'participation' and 'consultation'. Our conclusions are shown in *Table 5.4*.

Headteachers asked for further details about the role-playing activity. The following information was sent to participating schools.

Table 5.3. The sample of participating schools		
School	*No. of schools*	*No. children/young people*
Primary	10	604
Secondary	9	393
Total	19	997

In conversation with you and the young people we met in your school, we have decided to use role-play as one method to gather data for the Children and Young People's Health Project we discussed with you. Role-play is the means by which we can discover and understand what children/young people wish to tell us about what they feel are important aspects of seeking and receiving healthcare.

We will be asking each class of children/young people to work in small groups, to plan, and then act out, a short 5-minute role-play. Each group of children/young people will need to talk about and then choose a particular experience they wish to 'act out'. The sketch could take place, for example, in a particular healthcare setting, such as in a doctor's surgery, a clinic, a hospital, at home. The intention is to observe how they portray their experiences and then to ask them how and why they chose to portray them in this way. We will be looking for key messages that they would like to convey to us. We will avoid leading the children/young people. The role-play is about what they wish to tell us, not what we want to get answers to!

There will be no need for children/young people to write things down. Class teachers and/or classroom assistants may wish to make notes and share them with us afterwards. At the end of the activity we will take some time to check out, with the children/young people, that we have correctly understood the key messages they wanted to convey to us.

The whole activity will take up to one hour with each class. Reflective Learning-International staff, school nurses and the class teacher/classroom assistant are invited to be present at all times during the role-play.

We will negotiate a convenient time for us to visit you again after all concerned are satisfied that all appropriate ethical (consent) issues have been secured and all questions about this activity have been satisfactorily answered.

Role-play was a critical feature of this project. Role-play reflects issues about children and young people being free from pressure and manipulation, more specifically their right to express their views or, if they prefer, not to do

Table 5.4. The nature of participation in the Children and Young People's Project 2009–2010

Situation analysis	The situation analysis, i.e. recognition by senior PCT staff and school nurses of the need to know more about the experiences of 7–14 year-olds, in a large multi-cultural urban area, when accessing their health services.
Programme planning	A management decision was made to undertake the project through a school nursing service. The project design was co-constructed through discussion with healthcare professionals involved in the project schools and with children/young people.
Participation	*Implementation*: In implementing the project, the participatory methodology gave considerable power to children/young people. They acted as project 'shapers', researchers and active participants through role playing and cartoon drawing activities. In addition they organised themselves into 'conversation' and 'validation' groups for the purposes of project monitoring and evaluating outcomes. *Monitoring and evaluation*: Children/young people were involved in monitoring and evaluating the project. At all times classes and groups participated in the content and design of the technology-assisted tools. Children/young people met with appropriate adults throughout the project. They were involved in determining the criteria for evaluating the quality of the two tools. These were in the form of two sets of 'experiential metrics'.
Consultation	Children/young people were not simply asked for their views and experiences, they were actively involved throughout in shaping the content, methods and outcomes of the project. The outcomes were *by* them and *for* them.

so. Additionally, they should not be pressurised, constrained or influenced by adults, in ways that might prevent them from freely expressing their experiences of health services.

The number of different role-plays that were presented by the 680 children/ young people at this stage in the project, are shown in *Table 5.5*. The average size of the group presenting the role-play was 4-6.

Table 5.5. School role-plays

School	*Year group (in UK schools)*	*No. of children/ young people*	*No. of role play scenarios*
Primary	3, 4 and 5	407	77
Secondary	5, 6, 7, 8 and 9	273	49
Total		680	126

The general process of how we came to appreciate and understand children/ young people's experiences is shown in *Figure 5.1*.

The 126 role-plays provided a rich database for thematic analysis, and eventually, after an iterative process of (re)interpretation by and with the children and young people involved, two sets of experiential 'metrics' were derived. These are shown in *Figures 5.2 and 5.3*.

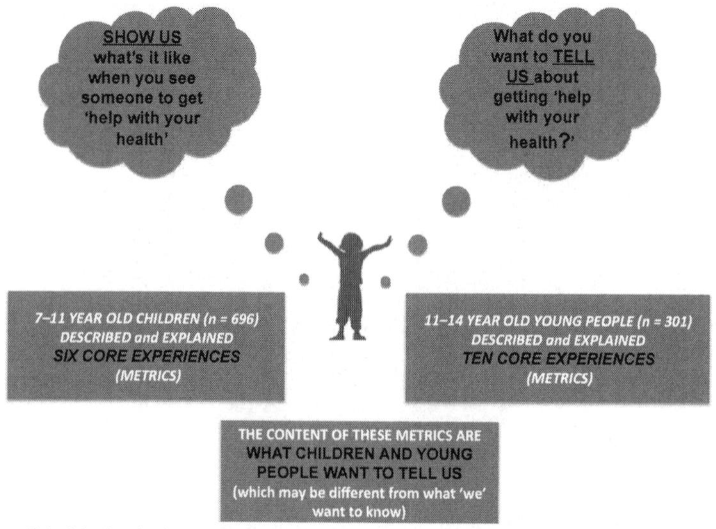

Figure 5.1. Methods that helped us appreciate and understand children and young people's experiences of health services.

SURROUNDINGS	The place was bright and colourful, with things to do while I waited.
ATMOSPHERE	People said and did things that helped create a calm atmosphere.
BEING FRIENDLY	People knew my name, said 'please', 'hello' and 'goodbye'.
COMFORTING	People reassured me, said everything would be ok and that I shouldn't be nervous.
UNDERSTANDING	People showed me that they really understood my problem.
CARING	People helped me cope with my problem and any pain.
LISTENING	People showed me that they were really listening to what I said and didn't rush me.
RESPECTING	I felt people respected me as a person and weren't bossy or pushy.
EXPLAINING	People talked to me in a way that I could understand, when asking questions and giving explanations.
WORTHWHILE	I felt I got something positive from the people I met.

Figure 5.2. The 10 experiential metrics from 11–14 year-old participants.

The children and young people involved in this project were asked to think about what they wanted the two technology-assisted 'tools' to look like. They were asked to think about the content and design. They came up with six 'design criteria. They wanted their tools to be:

- Technology-assisted, with a touch screen (not a paper-based tool).
- Visually 'appealing' on the screen, e.g. with smiley faces, cartoon characters.
- Not involving too much 'brain work'.
- Quick to complete.
- Including a scoring scale, e.g. 1–5.
- Where the content was 'theirs' and so reflected what they wanted to tell adults.

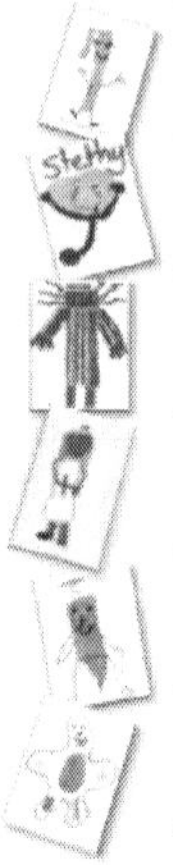

A NICE PLACE	A bright and colourful place with things to do while waiting
KNOWING WHAT HAPPENS	Knowing what happens when I get there
FRIENDLY PEOPLE	People smiling, saying I will be ok and that I will feel better soon
KIND PEOPLE	People using my name, saying hello, please and goodbye
CARING PEOPLE	People helping me to cope with pain (eg. a needle) and to be brave
GETTING A REWARD	Getting something (eg. lollipop, sticker) for going to the place

Figure 5.3. The six experiential metrics of 7–11 year-old participants.

Eventually these design criteria were transformed into two interactive, touch screen, multi-coloured tools. All the content including the question phrasing, the icons, the screen layout and colours came from the children and young people involved and were validated by them. *Figure 5.4* shows two of the 'pages' from the tool for 7–11 year-olds.

Some reflections

This was a challenging and significant project. There have been some notable achievements, but there is still a lot of unfinished business. One key thing we (re) learned was that children and young people can begin expressing their experiences of the health services they use from an early age, and we should not underestimate that. The challenge is to create safe spaces for them to freely express their views.

This capability to put gestures and words to experiences and to express themselves in non-verbal forms is just one side of the empowerment equation. The other involves adults' evolving capacity and willingness to listen to and learn from children and young people, to understand and consider their point of view, to be willing to re-examine their own opinions and attitudes and to envisage solutions that address children and young people's lived experiences. For all the adults involved in this project, as well as for the children and young people, participation was a challenging learning process and could not be reduced to a simple formula. Fulfilling the rights of children and young people to participate in (potentially)

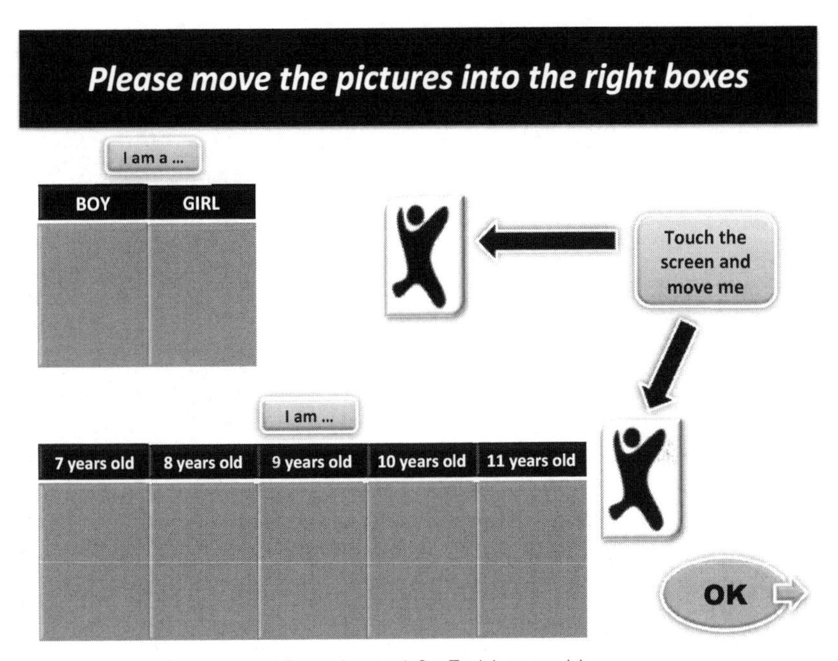

Figure 5.4. Two of the 'pages' from the tool for 7–11 year-olds.

empowering projects like this, where the outcomes were conceived and designed by the young people themselves, required many adults to reverse their thinking and practices. By this I mean a reversal from 'we' know best to 'they' know best. A reversal from this is what 'we' want to know, to this is what 'they' want to tell us.

Participation cannot be genuine if children and young people have no opportunity to understand the consequences and impact of their views and experiences on the quality and safety of health services for them. Non-genuine 'participation' merely disguises what is actually the manipulation of this age group of people to suit the needs and agendas of adults; to simply furnish adults with what adults want. This is tokenism, not the authentic participation of children and young people. The result is often disempowerment not empowerment. One important key to genuine participation is ensuring respect for children and young people's views.

In addition to facilitating and supporting appropriate activities that encouraged children and young people's participation in projects like this, it became increasingly clear to us that we had to do something meaningful and wise with what they were telling us. It was at this point in the project that all the rhetoric of empowerment through participation was most under pressure, it was when we began to realise what was truly at stake. There were two aspects to this. One was about integrity. By integrity I mean that as the project unfurled, it was obvious that expectations were being raised. The children and young people involved, as well as school staff and school nurses, were looking to see if what we said was what we were actually going to do. Put bluntly we had two fully validated interactive 'tools' ready for full implementation, comprising six metrics for 7–11 year-olds and 10 metrics for 11–14 year-olds, generated by children and young people themselves and for their use. So what were we going to do with them? A significant flaw in the project plan (see *Table 5.2*) was that it did not contain an implementation phase, just a design phase. So we had a problem. The second aspect was about strategy. Simply put, it was about how we were going to keep the momentum of the project going. How were we going to submit and gain approval, within the PCT, of an implementation phase at a time when the PCT was coping with the UK Health Secretary's announcement that Primary Care Trusts were to be abolished as part of a massive re-organisation of the NHS. In launching his White Paper, *Equity and excellence: Liberating the NHS* (Department of Health 2010), the Health Secretary said the coalition Government had initially expected PCTs to have a 'residual role'. In this White Paper, it stated that it was expected that PCTs, in the UK would cease to exist from April 2013. So politics and participation were colliding.

Three fickle friends

We learned that empowerment, participation and children and young people's rights can be an unsteady trio in several interesting ways. We value participation most when empowerment and rights come along with it. However, as we experienced in this project, even highly participatory approaches do not guarantee empowerment or the enactment of rights. So what did we think we did manage to achieve? *Tables 5.6 and 5.7* are an attempt to show some of the links between, and dimensions of, empowerment, participation and rights. The tables have been adapted from the work of Lansdown (2005).

If we think about the four dimensions of power, namely, power over, power with, power to, and power within, we gain a richer understanding of the project's achievements. The children and young people certainly achieved the power to design two highly innovative information-gathering tools. The opportunities that were created in the project meant that, to some extent, children and young people had power over those 'others' who normally determine whose knowledge is worth knowing. Taking part in the project added to the skills and self-confidence of the

Table 5.6. Measuring the quality of participation in the project 2009–2010	
Dimension	*Quality rating*
Ethical	*Excellent*: Children/young people were fully informed about the process and clear about the boundaries of what they were participating in. The interpretation of the views and experiences arising from the project, were checked and discussed with them. Consent was secured for each child/young person to participate in the project. They were free not to participate.
Child sensitive	*Excellent*: The adults involved used a range of creative strategies to allow children/young people to explore and express their ideas and experiences. Sufficient time was given to allow them to express themselves fully. School nurses, teachers and classroom assistants were all informed and involved in the day-to-day work of the project. The children/young people enjoyed the process and found many of the activities fun.
Voluntary and relevant	*Good*: Although the initiative did not arise from children's/young people's own expressed concerns, the aim of developing a process where they were able to authentically and confidentially express their experiences of health services was important and valued by them. The project was based on the importance of gathering their personal knowledge.
Inclusive	*Excellent*: The children/young people were drawn from different parts of the urban area to adequately represent the demographics of the city. They came from primary and secondary schools and were across the 7–14 age range. Girls and boys took part. All were treated with equal respect and were provided with opportunities to participate at levels appropriate to their capabilities.
Safe	*Excellent*: The project did not expose the children/young people to any risks. There was always an appropriate number of qualified adults in the room when project activities were being undertaken. All adults were checked by the Criminal Records Bureau.
Committed and sensitive staff	*Excellent*: The project leader was highly experienced and skilled in participatory techniques and committed to respect for children/young people's rights. All healthcare staff had expertise in the health of this age group.
Family and community links	*Excellent*: Parents (where appropriate) and school staff were consulted about whether their children could take part and were fully informed about the nature of the project.

Table 5.7. Impact of the project	
For children and young people	
Skills, understanding and knowledge	*Considerable impact:* The children/young people acquired a wide variety of ICT design skills and role-playing capabilities. They also had a better understanding of the links between themselves and their school nursing service. They reported that were proud of the two ICT-assisted tools that were developed and validated by them. Understanding of their own lived experiences of health services was dramatically enhanced through the iterative process of action and reflection.
Self-esteem and confidence	*Considerable impact:* The children/young people gained confidence in themselves as the project developed, both as a consequence of their enhanced skills, and through the experience of having their views listened to and respected.
Empowerment	*Considerable impact:* Due to the participatory and appreciative nature of the project, word spread that this was a very worthwhile activity. Groups of more experienced children/ young people in the project were empowering others.
Rights awareness	*Limited impact:* An implicit outcome was that the children/ young people realised that they were entitled to be taken seriously and respected and that they could positively influence the quality of health services for them.
Feeling that children/ young people had actually improved services	*No impact:* This was a highly problematic area. The project raised expectations but project workers were unable to give children/young people any clear statement about when their two ICT-assisted tools would be available across the city for all to use. This was both an implementation and strategic problem.
For school staff	
Participation	*Considerable impact:* School headteachers were delighted at being able to participate in the project. Class teachers and classroom assistants felt involved and interested in the project. Staff felt proud that their children/young people had been chosen to participate in the project.
Awareness of children/ young people's creative capacities	Staff were impressed by the level of skill the children/young people demonstrated in both cartoon creation and the design of the two ICT-assisted tools.

Table 5.7 (continued)	
Greater understanding of the importance of listening to children/young people	*Considerable impact*: Having observed the capacities of children/young people to participate, and seen the value that followed in gaining insight into how they experienced healthcare services and what was important to them, they were even more convinced of the importance of listening to and learning from the children/young people.
Greater respect for children/young people's rights	*Limited impact:* The project was not explicitly focused on promoting understanding of children/young people's rights. However, their right to be listened to and taken seriously emerged as a significant project outcome.
For local community health services	
Implementation and roll-out of two technology-assisted tools	*No impact:* To date, for financial and 'political' reasons (e.g. service re-organisation), the tools have not been used in any service settings (e.g. clinics, GP surgeries etc.).
Greater undertaking of what was in children/young people's best interests	*Considerable impact:* The findings from the project informed the School Nursing Services in the city. They had improved knowledge about children/young people's experiences of the services they delivered and managed, thus promoting the latter's best interests.
For the realisation of children/young people's rights	
Improved quality of services due to this project	*No impact:* To date there is no evidence of this.
Sustained commitment to respecting children/young people's right to participate in projects where their views and experiences are systematically gathered and fed back to healthcare professionals. This in turn to further develop and improve services for children/young people	*No impact:* To date there is no evidence of this.

participating individuals (power within). In observing the children and young people at work, the project seems to have added to their capacities to resolve disagreement, to learn from each other, to be creative, to be more confident in taking initiative and in negotiating with adults (power with). The impact of the project is shown in *Table 5.7*.

The fracture points in this project coalesced around implementation. Empowerment and the realisation of children and young people's rights are dependent on the nature and quality of participation. We discovered that it is perfectly possible for empowerment and rights realisation processes to be enhanced by 'agency' and frustrated by the surrounding 'opportunity structure'. Agency is the power children and young people have to shape their lives, make sense of their experiences, and influence decisions about their health. The opportunity structure is about the prospects for implementation and positive action. It is a highly political realm and comprises such things as the formal and informal 'rules of the game' which prescribe how, and by whom, decisions about implementation are to be made. The unity, strength and ideology of dominant groups form a second major aspect of this opportunity structure. In healthcare, as in many other areas, the wishes of subordinate groups can be blocked decisively by unity among powerful elites who are highly skilled at defending their positions of advantage and knowledge. A third aspect is an organisation's implementation capacity. In this project this was not so much to do with its administrative capacity but rather a significant policy change from central Government.

There is a fragility about participation: its difficulties in empowering the least powerful, its susceptibility to betrayal and truncation from outside and above. Some would finish this account by abandoning participation. But this strikes me as a fatalistic fairy-tale pretending that empowerment and children and young people's rights realisation can somehow be achieved without participation. Clearly clinicians and service leaders need to ensure that any work undertaken with children and young people will be worth while for the youngsters involved; that this will contribute to improving practices and so improve health services for children, young people and their families. Arguably without some serious consideration of the issues raised in this chapter, there is a danger that despite intensive input from children and young people, nothing will change and their time and energy will be wasted. There is the risk of facilitating the tokenistic involvement of children and young people, paying lip service, and reinforcing existing patterns that prevent this group from accessing quality health services.

References

Alderson P, Montgomery J (1996) *Health care choices: Making decisions with children.* Institute for Public Policy Research, London

Badham B (2002) Preface. In Willow C *Participation in practice: Children and young people as partners in change.* The Children's Society, London

Cartwright J, Crave S (2011) *Patient and public involvement toolkit.* BMJ Books, Wiley-Blackwell, Chichester

Department of Health (2004) National service framework for children, young people and maternity services: Executive summary. Department of Health, London

Department of Health (2005) *Creating a patient-led NHS: Delivering the NHS Improvement Plan.* Department of Health, London

Department of Health (2006) *You're welcome quality criteria self-assessment toolkit.* Department of Health, London

Department of Health and Department for Children, Schools and Families (2009) *Healthy lives, brighter futures – The strategy for children and young people's health.* Department of Health, London

Department for Children, Schools and Families (2008) *Every child matters outcomes framework.* HMSO, London

Department of Health and Department for Children, Schools and Families (2009) *Securing better health for children through world class commissioning. A guide to support delivery of Healthy lives, brighter futures: The strategy for children and young people's health.* HMSO, London

Department of Health (2010) *Equity and excellence: Liberating the NHS.* HMSO, London

House of Commons Health Committee (2007) *Patient and public involvement in the NHS. Third Report of Session 2006–07*, Volume 1. The Stationery Office, London

Lansdown G (2005) *Can you hear me? The right of young children to participate in decisions affecting them.* Working Paper 36. Bernard van Leer Foundation, The Hague, The Netherlands

Lavis P, Hewson L (2011) *How many times do we have to tell you? A briefing from the National Advisory Council About What Young People Think About Mental Health and Mental Health Services.* National Advisory Council, London

NHS Confederation (2011) *Children and young people's health – where next?* The NHS Confederation, London.

Robinson S (2010) Children and young people's view of health professionals in England. *Journal of Child Health Care* **14**(3): 310–26.

Royal College of Paediatrics and Child Health (RCPCH) (2010) *Not just a phase: A guide to the participation of children and young people in health services.* Royal College of Paediatrics and Child Health, London

United Nations (1989) *Convention on the rights of the child.* United Nations, Geneva

Worrall-Davies A (2008) Barriers and facilitators to children's and young people's views affecting CAMHS planning and delivery. *Child and Adolescent Mental Health* **13**(1): 16–18

YoungMinds (2011) *Talking about talking therapies: Thinking and planning about how best to make good and accessible talking therapies available to children and young people*. YoungMinds, London

Chapter 6

Empowering people with life-limiting conditions

Sue Lillyman and Heather Campbell

> *You matter because you are you.*
>
> (Cecily Saunders 1973)

Introduction

In this book there are many examples of empowering healthcare professionals, students and service users. In this chapter we review how we can empower people to remain in control of their care pathway when diagnosed with a life-limiting condition.

When people feel vulnerable and scared, such as when being diagnosed with a life-limiting condition, it might be more difficult from them to take control of their care (Mauksh et al 2008). In this chapter we review how people who have been diagnosed with such conditions can be empowered to have some control over their treatment and preferred place of care and death in relation to what Ghaye (2000) referred to as personal reality and developing a voice.

Background

Patients diagnosed with a life-limiting illness may not necessarily have a short time to live. A number of chronic conditions, including Parkinson's disease, multiple sclerosis and dementia, may have a long disease trajectory with slow decline over a number of years. By contrast patients diagnosed with motor neurone disease or aggressive or advanced cancers may have limited time where death may be foreseeable and inevitable. Palliative care is described by NICE (2004: 20) as:

> *The active holistic care of patients with advanced progressive illness. Management of pain and other symptoms and provision of psychological, social and spiritual support is paramount. The goal of palliative care is achievement of the best quality of life for patients and their families. Many aspects of palliative care are also applicable earlier in the course of the illness in conjunction with other treatments.*

Palliative care may be available at any stage of a patient's journey and may be part of a supportive care strategy for patients and families (NCPC 2006).

However it was the End of Life Care Strategy (Department of Health 2008a) that articulated the recognition that there was a particular need to identify those at end of life, acknowledging that as a patient's condition begins to deteriorate or a poor prognosis prevails, priorities and plans of care will by necessity change. Care and support should enable patient choice and control for all people nearing the end of their lives in all areas of the healthcare spectrum (National End of Life Care Programme 2009), not just for cancer patients receiving specialist palliative care. Therefore, all healthcare practitioners need to develop skills and knowledge in relation to empowering these patients to help them take more control over their care and treatment. In particular this may include having sensitive conversations about the future and plans for care, working as a team to meet care and treatment goals, respecting patient autonomy, choices and decisions, and supporting families pre- and post-death (Department of Health 2008a).

'No decision about me, without me' (Department of Health 2010: 3) has become part of the mantra for the NHS. However, when people are faced with life-limiting conditions they can often feel disempowered through not knowing what their options for care may be. They might have little understanding of their condition or feel confused and anxious about making any decisions about their care or treatment. The National Health Service End of Life Programme has produced a number of publications to assist patients and healthcare practitioners through the journey. These include, *Improving end of life care* (National End of Life Care Programme 2010a) and *Developing skills: Talking about end of life care* (National End of Life Care Programme 2010b).

As professionals it is our role to assist patients to be able to make informed decisions about their care and in this situation about their preferred place of care and death. The End of Life Strategy (Department of Health 2008a) and Lord Darzi in his publication, *NHS next stage review* (Department of Health 2008b), emphasised the need to give people more control and influence over their healthcare; this is never so important as when people are faced with life-limiting conditions. Through giving patients choice and a voice we can empower them to make decisions. However, we should avoid distress and stress where possible, and take into account patients' and families' wishes whilst maintaining clinical, cultural and ethical standards of care (Field and Cassel 2000).

It is also the patient's right to choose not to be involved either in decision making or receiving knowledge about their condition. As Toofany (2006) commented, empowerment cannot be given to the patient; the patient must want to be empowered. Therefore all people should be treated with respect by responding to their wishes and working with them to discover their preferred care pathway.

Difficult conversations

Paulo Freire, back in 1970, identified that one way to empower people is to have a mutual respect through dialogue. Drew et al (2001) and Frankel and Stein (1999) go on to suggest that the quality of the interaction between the patient and healthcare professional affects the success and outcome of healthcare provision. Effective conversations can result in increased satisfaction for the patient in relation to the care they receive (Koropchack et al 2006, McGuigan 2009, Uitterhoeve et al 2009). Hancock et al (2007) in their review also found that these conversations improved end of life care and Murray et al (2006) noted that such conversations engender hope for the patient.

The General Medical Council (2010) advocates working in partnership with patients, respecting their rights and wishes to reach decisions in relation to their personal treatment and care. Other healthcare professionals' codes of conduct also echo the need for respect, care and dignity of all patients (Nursing and Midwifery Council 2008, Health Professions Council 2008). However, even with these in place the National End of Life Care Programme (2010c) still found that the complaints received from people at the end of life related to breakdown in communication between staff/relatives and patients and poor staff attitudes. Communication was also found as a major issue in hospital complaints by the National Audit Office (2008) and National Confidential Enquiry into Patient Outcome and Death (2009).

When receiving test results, a prognosis or other upsetting news it can be a hard time for the patient, the family and the healthcare professional, it is also one of the most difficult times to have a conversation with the people involved However, Tapp (2001) noted that making the space for these conversations may result in giving patients the opportunity of making sense of their illness and suffering. Lillyman and Campbell (2011) discuss how we can approach these conversations and the importance of listening to patients, setting their agenda for the conversations and developing skills in picking up cues from the patient throughout. Frankel and Stein (1999) identify the importance of the healthcare professional investing in the beginning of the conversation with the patient. Initiating these conversations may present the professional with concerns about time and workload; however, Langewitz et al (2002) introduced the 90-second dialogue as an aid to eliciting the patient's agendas for these conversations.

England (2005) suggested that a well-honed conversation is an expression of critical thinking, communication and intervention skills that are indispensable in the delivery of patient-focused care. It is therefore important that when engaged in these conversations the healthcare professional observes how the patient reacts to the conversations in particular situations, and their own reactions to the conversation (McGuigan 2009). Each conversation is unique, and reflecting on conversations helps practitioners to develop conversational skills, to become sensitive to patients' cues, to identify patients' agendas and to empower patients to take control over their care journey (Lillyman and Campbell 2011). Clayton et al (2008) also found that patients and their carers mostly preferred honest and accurate information from their healthcare professional; this they suggest should be given with empathy and understanding. Uitterhoeve et al (2009) also identify the importance of responding to cues as these are often indications of worries or concerns.

Wright and Leahey (2000) go on to suggest that it is the nurses' attitudes that are the key element in establishing a relationship and trust at the beginning of the conversation. Weiner and Efferen (2005) and Mauksch et al (2008) state that the healthcare professional should have a good pre-existing relationship and rapport with the patient as well as professional clinical experience and good recognition of the severity and chronicity of the illness the person is suffering from. McGuigan (2009) highlights the importance of placing the patient at the centre of the conversation. Mauksch et al (2008) identify that the conversation should include up-front agenda setting and acknowledgement of social or emotional cues. These are discussed later in this chapter.

Barriers to effective communication may come from the healthcare professional who feels unprepared for such conversations. Healthcare professionals might fear making things worse for the patient and be afraid of unleashing strong emotions and facing their own failure (National End of Life Programmes 2011a). They might even use distracting techniques. Barriers can also come from the patient in not wanting to be a burden to the health staff (National End of Life Programmes 2011a) or, at this time, not being ready for the conversation.

Conversations therefore need to be addressed at an appropriate time for the patient and healthcare professional, conducted with sensitivity and respect and handled in a professional manner.

Making decisions for end of life care

With a diagnosis of a life-limiting illness or if the patient is in the final stages of life there might seem little point in discussing empowerment. However, this is an important time for patients, their carers and families and there is every need to engage patients in making decisions in relation to their preferred care plan.

One of the seven principles in the National End of Life Programme (2009) is that the choices and priorities of individual patients remain central to any plan and delivery of care and their wishes and beliefs are paramount in all decision making. Many Government and professional documents remind us of the need to support patients to make these decisions at this stage, including the End of Life Care Strategy (Department of Health 2008a) and various publications from the NHS National End of Life Strategy Care Programme (2009, 2010a, 2010b, 2010c, 2010d). Besides verbally stating their preferences there are a number of options available to assist patients to record their wishes. This can be through recording an advance care plan or through appointing a lasting power of attorney to make decisions for them once they have lost capacity to make decisions themselves.

A further aspect of care according to the Kings Fund (2011) is that patients should be given as much control over their environment as possible to provide privacy, respect and comfort at this time of their life.

Advance care plans: Statement and decisions

Empowerment can be given to patients through knowledge, either about their condition, the services available or choices of treatment and care. This will enable patients to make advance plans for end of life care while they still have the capacity to do so.

This process of advance care planning is a voluntary ongoing discussion which should be reviewed frequently and recorded. The Government and other organisations have produced a number of documents and guidelines to assist people to make and record their choices, wishes and decisions.

Under the Mental Capacity Act (MCA) 2005 there are three ways of expressing outcomes of advance care planning discussions.

Advance statement

An advance statement is the written or expressed wishes of a patient declaring what they would or would not like to happen in the event of their condition deteriorating and capacity being lost (National End of Life Care Programme 2010d, 2011a). This might include where they wish to be cared for and die, their funeral choices, etc. Although not legally binding it should have legal standing and where at all possible be taken into consideration by carers when making decisions. It should be noted that treatments and specific interventions may also be requested by patients but may not be agreed to by medical staff if it is not in the best interests of the patient.

Advance decisions

An advance decision to refuse treatment is a legally binding declaration of a patient's choice to refuse certain treatments, some of which may be life-sustaining, in anticipation of how their condition may affect them in the future when they may not have the capacity to make these decisions themselves (National End of Life Care Programme 2011b). Advance decisions were previously known as advance directives or living wills.

Murray et al (2006) note that an advance decision may be a written document that involves informed consent for the refusal of specific treatments. Advance decisions are made voluntarily when the person has capacity to do so (National End of Life Care Programme 2011b).

An advance decision should specify the treatments the patient wishes to refuse and the specific circumstances in which it applies. When such a decision involves life-sustaining treatment it should be documented, signed and witnessed and include the statement 'even if my life is at risk' (MCA 2005). It cannot include the refusal of any basic comfort or care measures (End of Life Care Programme and National Council for Palliative Care 2008). It may however include refusal of the following: antibiotics for an infection, use of percutaneous endoscopic gastrostomy (PEG) or any other means of artificial nutrition and hydration, mechanical ventilation or any form of resuscitation should breathing or heart fail. For an advance decision to refuse treatment to be applicable and valid it should fulfil certain criteria and if deemed to be valid must be followed (End of Life Care programme and National Council for Palliative Care 2008).

A dialogue that is open and that includes forward planning should be encouraged when a patient has strong beliefs in relation to any life-sustaining treatment or preferences for care (British Medical Association 2009). These issues should be discussed with a healthcare professional who knows the patient's particular health circumstances.

Until capacity is lost patients should be encouraged to participate and engage in any decision making involving their care and treatment. Healthcare professionals should also discuss with patients their right to change their mind, whilst they still have capacity, at any stage even after an advance statement or decision has been made.

In summary, any advance care plan, statement or directive should include important information about the patient's concerns, values and preferences (National End of Life Programmes 2009). Although healthcare professionals should provide opportunities and take the lead in initiating these conversations they should be voluntary, approached with sensitivity, and not undertaken at the point of diagnosis.

Lasting power of attorney

Some people may not want to write their preferences for care within an advance care statement, or may feel they are unable to make such decisions in relation to their preferred care. A further option is to appoint another person as a lasting power of attorney. This is where a patient appoints a person to make decisions on his or her behalf, once again only when the patient has lost capacity to do so him or herself. This process is completed through a solicitor and can be given for financial and/or health issues. Here individuals do not write their preferences but chose someone who they trust to make their wishes known should they not be able to do so themselves.

Duhamel and Dupius (2004) acknowledge the existence and expertise of family and unpaid carers and Briggs (2010) also noted the importance of having an increased awareness of the carer and family dynamics and their experiences. It is important to know and work with carers and families who might have other points of view than the patient. Carers and family members might want to keep their loved one alive longer, while the patient may have strong feelings about not receiving life-sustaining treatment should the situation arise. Krumberger (2003) reminds us that each point of view is valid and that they should be acknowledged.

Best interests of the patient and empowerment

Some patients may not have specific wishes or requests in relation to their end of life care. However, there is a need to continue to treat these patients with respect, dignity and sensitivity, and where decisions are left to healthcare professionals they must be in the 'best interests' of the patient. The patient should still be encouraged to participate in any decision (National End of Life Care programme 2010d). Briggs (2010) notes the importance of providing opportunities to discuss personal needs and preferences at every stage of care and treatment. Assumptions should always be avoided; even if a patient has no preferences in one aspect of care, he or she may have preferences about other aspects and therefore should be consulted throughout.

The healthcare practitioners' role in empowerment

Health professionals can be viewed as being in a position of power in relation to their knowledge and role as caregiver. They are also in a position to assist and encourage patients to gain control over their own lives (Grace 1991). Empowerment, on many occasions, might mean a shift from the professional knowing best, to supporting and empowering patients to be in control of their wishes, including the right to change their minds about what they want.

Nurses' and healthcare professionals' power, according to Benner (1984), includes advocacy and problem solving powers. Acting as an advocate enables patients' views and preferences to be known and helps them to gain a voice in their care. Nurses and health professionals can assist patients to take control and ownership of their care.

Conversations with patients can evoke strong emotions as sensitive issues may be discussed. Healthcare professionals may avoid emotions so as not to damage the patient (Sheldon et al 2006, Bratass et al 2009) or themselves (Gordon et al 2009). However, difficult emotions should be acknowledged and the appropriate support provided. Because of the multi-professional approach of palliative care this may be from a spiritual advisor, psychologist, counsellor or social worker (Duhamel and Dupius 2004). Before taking on these conversations, Krumberger (2003) suggests that as healthcare professionals we need to review our own feelings and position at the time. McGuigan (2009) also advises preventing misunderstanding and unrealistic expectations, and suggests that healthcare professionals should draw on their advanced communication skills. These skills include summarising and reflecting on the discussion, looking for cues, building a good rapport, using mindful practice and maintaining a focus on the patient's agenda (Lillyman and Campbell 2011). The National End of Life Programme (2009) also includes the use of active listening, legitimisation of patients' views, valuing knowledge, and experience of their needs.

Murray et al (2006) also highlight the importance of providing realistic information in a sensitive manner whilst maintaining feelings of normality and giving patients time to develop new coping strategies.

Support

Support is particularly important for those staff who engage in these difficult conversations. However the National End of Life Programme (2011) notes that there is a lack of support in this situation for healthcare professionals. Support should be sought through formal or informal clinical supervision to help the health professional deal with these difficult conversations (Lillyman 2007). Clinical supervision should include critical reflection on the experience and the development of action plans, which will make health professionals better able to deliver informed knowledge-based care when faced with a similar situation (Johns 2004).

Conclusion

As suggested earlier some patients have strong wishes for their end of life care provision, others not. Empowerment is about helping all patients with as many decision making opportunities as they want. It is not to force people to take control but rather to keep them informed at every stage of their condition and to revisit their wishes frequently. Any of the above provision, including advance care plans and the appointment of a lasting power of attorney, only come into place once patients have lost the capacity to make decisions for themselves. Patients may change their minds at any stage.

In summary we quote Cecily Saunders (1967)

> *When we look back we remember not what death has done for them but what they have done to our thoughts about it.*

Points for reflection

The following issues were raised within this chapter.

- Patients at the end of life may well feel vulnerable and disempowered.
- Communication is a way of empowering patients to have some control over their care journey.
- There are a variety of processes that patients can be encouraged to engage in when they still have capacity, to ensure their wishes and preferences are carried out when possible.
- Self-empowerment is possible when facing life-limiting conditions and at the end of life.

References

Benner P (1984) *From novice to expert.* Addison-Wesley, California

Bratass H, Thorsnes S, Hargie O (2009) Cancer nurses narrating after conversations with cancer outpatients. How do nurses' roles and patients' perspectives appear in the nurses' narratives? *Scandinavian Journal of Caring Science* **23**: 767–74

Briggs D (2010) Notes on end of life; the social interactions between patients, carers and professionals. *Quality and Ageing and Older Adults* **11**(2): 35–46

British Medical Association (2009) *End of life decisions.* BMA, London

Clayton JM, Hancock K, Parker S et al (2008) Sustaining hope when communicating with terminally ill patients and their families: A systemic review. *Psychooncology* **17** (7): 641–59

Department of Health (2005) *Mental Capacity Act.* The Stationery Office, London

Department of Health (2008a) *End of life strategy: Promoting high quality care for all adults at the end of life.* The Stationery Office, London

Department of Health (2008b) *NHS next stage.* The Stationery Office. London

Department of Health (2010) *Equity and excellence. Liberating the NHS.* The Stationery Office, London

Drew P, Chatwin J, Collins S (2001) Conversations analysis: A method for research into interactions between patients and health care professionals. *Health Expectations* **4**: 58–70

Duhamel F, Dupuis F (2004) Guaranteed returns: Investing in a conversation with families of patients with cancer. *Clinical Journal of Oncology Nursing* **8**(1): 68–71

England M (2005) Analysis of nurse conversation: Methodology of the process recording. *Journal of Psychiatric and Mental Health Nursing* **12**: 661–71

Field MJ, Cassel CK (2000) *Approaching death: Improving care at end of life.* (2nd edn) National Academy Press, Washington DC

Frankel EM, Stein T (1999) Getting the most out of the clinical encounter: The four habits model. *Permanente Journal* **3**(3): 70–88

Freire P (1970) *Pedagogy of the oppressed.* Continuum Publishing Company, New York

General Medical Council (2010) *Treatment and care towards the end of life. Good practice in decision making.* GMC, London

Ghaye T (2000) Empowerment through reflection: Is this a case of the emperor's new clothes? In Ghaye T, Gillespie D, Lillyman S (eds) *Empowerment through reflection.* (pp 65–91) Quay Books, Dinton

Gordon C, Ellis-Hill C, Ashburn A (2009) The use of conversational analysis: Nurse patient interaction in communication disability after stroke. *Journal of Advanced Nursing* **65**(3): 544–53

Grace V (1991) The marketing of empowerment and the construction of the health consumer; a critique of health promotion. *International Journal of Health Studies* **21**(2): 329–43

Hancock K, Clayton JM, Parker SM et al (2007) Truth telling in discussing prognosis in advanced life-limiting illness: A systematic review. *Palliative Medicine* **21**(6): 507–17

Health Professional Council (2008) *Standards of conduct, performance and ethics*. HPC, London

Johns C (2004) *Becoming a reflective practitioner* (2nd edn). Blackwell Publishing, Oxford

Kings Fund (2011) *Routes to success in end of life care: Achieving quality environments for end of life*. The Kings Fund, London

Koropchack CM, Pollack KI, Arnold RM et al (2006) Studying communication in oncologist–patient encounters. The SCOPE trial. *Palliative Medicine* **20**: 813–19

Krumberger J (2003) Difficult conversations. *RN* **66**(11): 2–3

Langewitz W, Denz M, Keller A et al (2002) Spontaneous talking time at the start of consultations in outpatient clinic: Cohort study. *British Medical Journal* **325**: 682–3

Lillyman S (2007) What clinical supervision means. In Lillyman S, Ghaye T (eds) *Effective clinical supervision: The role of reflection* (2nd edn) Quay Books, London

Lillyman S, Campbell H (2011) Difficult conversations: Discussing what matters. In Ghaye T, Lillyman S (eds) *When caring is not enough* (pp 45–56) Mark Allen Publishers, Dinton

Mauksch LB, Dugdale DC, Dodson S, Epstein R (2008) Relationship, communication and efficiency in the medical encounter. *Archives of Internal Medicine* **168**(13): 1387–95

McGuigan D (2009) Communicating bad news to patient: A reflective approach. *Nursing Standard* **23**(31): 51–6

Murray SA, Sheikh A, Thomas K (2006) Advance care planning in primary care: Uncomfortable but likely to engender hope rather than dispel it. *British Medical Journal* **333**: 868–9

National Audit Office (2008) *Feeding back? Learning from complaints handling in health and social care*. The Stationery Office, London

National Confidential Enquiry into Patient Outcome and Death (2009) *Caring to the End? A review of the care of patients who died in hospital within four days of admission*. National Confidentially Enquiry into Patient Outcome and Death, London

National Council for Palliative Care (NCPC) (2006) *Paliaitive care explained*. NCPC, London.

National End of Life Care Programme and National Council for Palliative Care (2008) *Advance decisions to refuse treatment, A guide for health and social care*. Professionals National End of Life Care Programme, London

National End of Life Care Programme, Skills for Health, Skills for Care and Department of Health (2009) *Common core competences and principles for health and social care workers working with adults at the end of life to support End of Life Care Strategy*. National End of Life Care Programme, London

National End of Life Care Programme, Skills for Health, Skills for Care and Department of Health (2010a) *Improving end of life care*. National End of Life Care Programme, Leicester

National End of Life Care Programme, Skills for Health, Skills for Care and Department of Health (2010b) *Developing skills: Talking about end of life*. National End of Life Care Programme, London

National End of Life Care Programme (2010c) *An Analysis of the numbers of hospital complaints relating to End of Life care over a six month period.* National End of Life Care Programme. London

National End of Life Care Programme (2010d) *Advanced care planning support sheet 3.* National End of Life Care Programme, London

National End of Life Care Programme (2011a) *Finding the words*. National End of Life Care Programme, London

National End of Life Care Programme (2011b) *Capacity, care planning and advance care planning in life limiting illness*. National End of Life Care Programme, London

National Institute for Health and Clinical Excellence (NICE) (2004) *Cancer service guidance: Improving supportive and palliative care for adults with cancers: The manual.* NICE, London

Nursing and Midwifery Council (2008) *The Code; Standards of conduct, performance and ethics for nurses and midwives.* NMC, London

Saunders C (1967) The care of terminal stages of cancer. *Annals of the Royal College of Surgeons of England* **41**(Sppl 1) 162–9

Saunders C (1973) Death in the family: A professional view. *British Medical Journal* **1**: 30–1

Sheldon LK, Barrett R, Ellington L (2006) Difficult conversations in nursing. *Journal of Nursing Scholarship* **38**(2): 141–7

Tapp DM (2001) Conserving the validity of suffering: Addressing family constraints to illness conversation. *Nursing Inquiry* **8**(4): 254–63

Toofany S (2006) Patient empowerment: Myth or reality? *Nursing Management* **13**(6): 18–22

Uitterhoeve R, Bensing J, Diven E, Donders R, deMulder P, Achterberg T (2009) Nurse–patient communication in cancer care: Does responding to patient's cues predict patient satisfaction with communication? *Psychooncology* **18**: 1060–8

Weiner JS, Efferen LS (2005) Recognition and communication. *Chest* 127(6): 1886–8

Wright LM, Leahey M (2000) *Nurses and families: A guide to family assessment and intervention* (3rd edn) FA Davies, Philadelphia

Chapter 7

Empowering students through the use of storyboarding

Sue Lillyman and Clare Bennett

Introduction

The learner is not an empty vessel to be filled, but a flame to be ignited.
Defo from Plato (427–347 BC)

Empowerment of students in the classroom is pivotal in allowing individuals to flourish. Through facilitating empowerment value is added to the learning encounter. Learning becomes dynamic, the process is opened up, situations are seized and, importantly, acted upon (Ghaye 2011).

In this chapter we explore storyboarding as an approach to engendering empowerment in the classroom setting. In using storyboarding a conscious decision is made by educators to use a positive approach to reflection by assisting students to amplify what they can do and what they know, rather than taking a problem-based approach to education. Storyboarding provides students with the opportunity to share and celebrate their lived experience with their peers. It provides space for deeper reflection on practice and allows for learning from lived experiences to be reflected upon within the classroom environment.

Empowering students in the classroom

Empowerment through teaching is underpinned by a partnership between the educator and student in achieving a shared vision. It is characterised by a humanistic approach based on feminist values which promote a culture of nurturing, caring, growth and support (Chally 1992). Petersen et al (2008) argue that empowerment is not a theory but a philosophy. Campbell (2003) identified it as an exchange that happens at various times; it is a continuous and ever-changing process that occurs throughout life.

Espeland and Shanta (2001) highlight that educators cannot empower students if they are encouraged to adopt the role of passive recipient, for example through staff decreasing their expectations or taking the responsibility for learning away from them. Instead, the student has to commit to the empowerment process.

In order to capture this approach to learning and teaching and to empower students in the classroom then the old patriarchal world view of education should be avoided. Instead, a shared vision of education between educators and students needs to be developed. Storyboarding can facilitate this shared vision approach by acknowledging and valuing students' beliefs, experiences and concerns, in a positive manner, in order to help them shape a successful outcome (Cederbaum and Klusaritz 1999).

History of storyboarding

Storyboarding, according to Lottier (1986), is attributed to Leonardo Da Vinci and was adapted by Walt Disney and the film industry who used the approach when developing stories for new films (Barnes 1996). Lottier (1986) also identified its use more recently in the business world to form action plans. Cox (2008) introduced storyboarding into education when assisting students to develop health promotion messages for television. Recently it has been introduced into healthcare education (Ghaye et al 2008, Lillyman and Bennett 2010, Lillyman et al 2011).

In the early stages of using storyboarding, an emphasis was placed on the creation of stories and plans. However, when applied to healthcare education, the emphasis is on lived experiences. It focuses on bringing those in the classroom to share and reflect on their practice in order to learn from these experiences.

Storytelling and narrative

Storyboarding is an extension of storytelling and narratives, which also have an important role in the classroom. Levett-Jones (2007:13) defines narratives as

> *....a brief recount of an actual situation or episode in clinical practice that is significant because it resulted in new learning and/or new understanding.*

Narrative on its own can be absorbing, it engages listeners and invites them to make an interpretation of the situation (Greenhalgh and Hurwitz 2009). However, it is not concerned with just telling a story because it is interesting, demanding or exciting. Instead, the story relates to an event that captures lived experiences that can then be systematically reflected on and analysed.

Storytelling and narratives are not always recognised in Western society as a valid way of passing on information and knowledge. However, Newman (2003) found that the brain seems built to process stories rather than other forms of input and found that people respond strongly to stories and identify them as a useful way of learning. Storytelling can create an enhanced deeper and broader understanding of practice and theory and can, therefore, be a vehicle for change in the future (Petersson et al 2009). Bringing knowledge and practice together through meaningful dialogue can promote interpretive analysis and reflection (Rittman and Stella 1995).

Narratives and storytelling have been widely used in medical and health education (Newman 2003). Spouse (2003) used narrative and storytelling with her student nurses and found that it helped the students to reframe their self-image and develop further professional understanding. As Levett-Jones (2007) points out, it provides an opportunity to uncover nursing practices that often go unnoticed. It can also provide extra information and different perspectives of the situation through group discussion (Greenhalgh and Hurwitz 2009).

Therefore, through critical reflection on the story, students, with their colleagues and facilitators, can critically review their practice. They can develop an understanding of how they work that is based on a firm knowledge base, with a view to refinement and improvement of and/or, if appropriate, a change in their approach to care.

Empowering students through storytelling

Hawkins and Lindsay (2006) identified the importance of storytelling, arguing that an individual's experiences cannot be captured in any textbook. These they note are real experiences for the student who has lived through them. Although knowledge is often seen as the key to empowerment, Chally (1992) emphasises the power of inclusion that comes through coalition and building with others. Through this sharing of the experience in the classroom, Levett-Jones (2007) suggests that storytelling goes beyond the description of the experience to in-depth analysis and reflection on the episode which, in turn, assists students to critique, develop critical competence, learn from and value their practice. Additionally, students can make sense of their practice through storytelling (Hunter 1991). By affirming their stories in the classroom a positive message is given to students in relation to their practice and learning through a shared vision (Chally 1992).

Ghaye (2011) asserts that making sense of and attributing meaning normally occurs in a social context. The classroom can, therefore, be an appropriate place for this process. Ghaye et al (2008) refer to the process as 'collective wisdom' where other students can reflect on and analyse the story, thereby gaining further insight into the theory and practice of the clinical arena.

Storyboarding

The storyboarding approach encourages students to use the right side of the brain, which is associated with creativity, as well as the left side, which is known as the 'thinking' side (Starbuck 2006). It is also a good way of stimulating effective theoretical learning and group critical reflection through sharing of experiences (Lillyman et al 2011).

When using storyboarding in the classroom setting the educator is the facilitator of the session and identifies the subject area for the session. For example, it might be based on end of life care, communication issues, caring for a patient with a specific illness, etc. The session then requires students to identify an experience that they feel confident about sharing with their peers within the classroom. It relies on them recalling an event and their ability to tell their peers what happened.

Once students have their story, based on the session subject, they work in groups of up to eight people. Smaller groups can work in pairs. All the students in the small group are encouraged to share their story with the rest of their peers in that group. At this point they begin to engage in critical conversations and develop Ghaye et al's (2008) 'collective wisdom', as noted above, through a coherent integration of the diverse issues that are unearthed. By working together, the diversity of outputs is much greater than any individual would generate alone. Kemp (2009) also used the creation of collective empowerment when she brought midwives together to share their views and experiences through theatre.

Once all the stories are shared in their small groups, there is an opportunity for each group to choose one story that they will adopt as a group story, complete the storyboard and present it to the whole class for discussion. At this stage the students are asked to write and draw their stories in a series of six stages. Through this process the student is able to rearrange ideas and start to put them into a pattern or sequence (Lottier 1986). By drawing and writing the storyboard the students are able to affirm their stories.

As Hawkins and Lindsey (2006) noted, committing the story to writing, or in this case drawing, is more powerful than just talking since it stays on the page and does not dissipate over time. It also provides students with space and time to rehearse and make sense of their story. This can help the student develop critical thinking through the process of questioning and sequential thinking (Fornis and Penden-McAlpine 2007).

Once the storyboards are completed they are placed around the room for the wider group to view. The final stage involves students telling their stories to their peers in the larger group and the facilitator assisting with summarising, reviewing, reflecting and assisting the students to relate theory to their practice. The facilitator also needs to identify any emerging themes. This collaborative learning experience leads to mutual growth for the student and the facilitator (Cederbaum and Klusaritz 2009).

Empowering students through storyboarding

Although the process of using narratives and storytelling is powerful in itself (Spouse 2003), by creating storyboards students can rearrange their ideas into a pattern or sequence before stepping back to reflect and again rearrange their thoughts. Espeland and Shanta (2001) propose that as these stories and experiences are shared, the process can itself lead to a sense of empowerment for the students. They go on to suggest that by allowing students to participate in their education, their learning has the potential to become more rewarding and exciting. Through this approach there is also an increase in self-esteem and political skills for the student (Lillyman et al 2011).

Using the storyboarding approach in the classroom, particularly with healthcare students, can lead to a dichotomy for healthcare educators between the aims of the industry, i.e. producing a safe, knowledgeable practitioner, and a humanistic approach to learning (Espeland and Shanta 2001). However, if the students' experiences are valued, the facilitator can guide the reflections and critical analysis to produce a safe and effective practitioner through the application of theory into practice. Schreiber and Banister (2002) refer to this as emancipatory education. Student empowerment in this situation is, therefore, through collaborative learning and mutual growth (Cederbaum and Klusaritz 2009).

Facilitating the process

Nurse education is effective when it includes a positive correlation between theoretical learning and practical application (Steen and Costello 2008). As Darbyshire and Flemming (2008) identify, education is a complex space and should not be confined to lectures. This caution is echoed by Campbell (2003), who notes that educators can easily fall prey to the pressures of moving students through the set educational programme with the end result of depositing them into practice. However, by giving students autonomy in the classroom, educators can incorporate Foucault's approach of student empowerment (Darbyshire and Flemming 2008). In addition, by adopting a pedagogical and strengths-based approach to adult learning, students can feel empowered in situations where they may otherwise feel powerless or lack the appropriate skill capacity (Cederbaum and Klusaritz 2009). Through this approach students can be encouraged to think differently, to become more self-directed and develop into reflective practitioners. It can also assist students in their self-discovery and development of a capacity to control and take responsibility for their own learning (Petersen et al 2008).

However, using this approach involves students having to relive their experiences in front of their peers, as noted above, which can potentially cause some concern if it is not facilitated sensitively. Van Manen (1990) highlights the vulnerability of students when they are dealing with sensitive issues such as care of the dying patient, emphasising the need for supportive facilitation throughout these sessions. As Levett-Jones and Bourgeois (2007) pointed out, sharing lived experiences can lead to tensions between what students do and do not know, and what they can and cannot do. The facilitator also needs to be aware of the danger of focusing on the simplicity of the situation and the potential to neglect more complex considerations (Newman 2003). Facilitators also need to be experts in the field that is being presented and identify their own limitations.

Myrick and Tamlyn (2007) identified that using storyboarding can venture outside the educator's comfort zone and may give rise to some uncertainty, ambiguity and frustration. It can even be painful according to Levett-Jones (2007), whilst at the same time meaningful and memorable. Newman (2003) notes that powerful memory stimuli are an important means to transmit cultural identity, norms and traditions. Whilst positive in promoting learning, storyboarding may give rise to sensitive issues that need addressing in a positive manner within the classroom.

This emancipatory approach to teaching helps to develop critical reflection on which students can create their own meaning through engaging with others through dialogue (Schreiber and Banister 2002). According to Campbell (2003) the facilitation of the empowering experience should be consciously made by those in the role of educating the student. A strengths perspective approach can support this where an emphasis is placed on discovery, affirmation, capabilities, interests, knowledge, resources, goals and objectives (Cederbaum and Klusaritz 2009).

Conclusions

Storyboarding helps students to link together knowledge and practice through a meaningful dialogue, interpretive analysis and reflection (Levett-Jones 2007). Through this approach to education the student can be empowered and transformed into a safe and knowledgeable practitioner (Lauterbach and Hertz 2005). This can be created through a shared vision between the student and educator/facilitator (Chally 1992) and result in an autonomous student and practitioner.

Points for reflection

The following issues have been raised in this chapter:

- Empowerment cannot be given to students; both the student and educator must commit to the process.
- There is often a struggle between the educator's requirement of the curriculum and engagement in autonomous student learning.
- Reflecting on real lived experience can result in producing a safe and knowledgeable practitioner.
- There is a need to readdress the power relationship between the student and the educator.

References

Barnes MD (1996) Using storyboarding to determine components of wellness for university students. *Journal of American College Health* **44**(4): 180

Campbell S (2003) Cultivating empowerment in nursing today for a strong profession tomorrow. *Journal of Nursing Education* **42**(9): 423–6

Cederbaum J, Klusaritz HA (2009) Clinical instruction; using the strengths based approach with nursing students. *Journal of Nursing Education* **48**(8): 422–8

Chally P (1992) Empowerment through teaching. *Journal of Nursing Education* **31**(3): 117–20

Cox C (2008) 'Good for you TV': Using storyboarding for health-related television public service announcement to analyze message and influence positive health choices. *Journal of School Health* **78**(3): 179–83

Darbyshire C, Fleming V (2008) Mobilizing Foucault: History, subjectivity and autonomous learners in nurse education. *Nursing Inquiry* **15**(4): 263–9

Espeland K, Shanta L (2001) Empowering verses enabling in academia. *Journal of Nursing Education* **40**(8): 342–6

Fornis S, Peden-McAlpine C (2007) Evaluation of a reflective learning intervention to improve critical thinking in novice nurses. *Journal of Advanced Nursing* **57**(4): 410–21

Ghaye T (2011)*Teaching and learning through reflective practice. A practical guide for positive actions* (2nd edn) Routledge, London

Ghaye T, Melander-Wikman A, Kisare M, Chambers P, Ulrika B, Kostenius C, Lillyman, S (2008) Participatory and appreciative action and reflection (PAAR) democratizing reflective practices. *Reflective Practice* **9**(4): 361–98

Greenhalgh T, Hurtwitz B (2009) Narrative based medicine: Why study narrative? *British Medical Journal* **318**: 48–50

Hawkins J, Lindsey E (2006) We listen but do we hear? The importance of patient stories. *British Journal of Community Nursing* **11**(9): 56–64

Hunter KM (1991) *Doctors' stories: The narrative structure of medical knowledge.* Princeton University Press, Princeton, NJ

Kemp J (2009) Exploring empowerment issues with student midwives using forum theatre. *British Journal of Midwifery* **17**(7): 438–9

Lauterbach SS, Hentz PB (2005) Journaling to learn: A strategy in nurse education for developing the nurse as person and person as nurse. *International Journal for Human Caring* **9**(1): 29–35

Levett-Jones T (2007) Facilitating reflective practice and self-assessment of competence through the use of narratives. *Nurse Education in Practice* **7**: 112–19

Levett-Jones T, Bourgeois S (2007) *The clinical placement: An essential guide for nursing student.* Elsevier, Sydney

Lillyman S, Bennett C (2010) Using storyboarding approach to develop critical thinking based on students lived experiences. *Worcester Journal of Learning and Teaching.* Available from: at http://worc.ac.uk/adpu/documents/extabsractsslillyman.pdf.

Lillyman S, Gutteridge R, Berridge P (2011) Using a storyboarding technique in the classroom to address end of life experiences in practice and engage student nurses in deeper reflection. *Nurse Education in Practice* **11**(3): 179–85

Lottier LF (1986) Storyboarding your way to successful training. *Public Personal Management* **15**(4): 421–7

Myrick F, Tamlyn D (2007) Teaching can never be innocent: Fostering an enlightening education experience. *Journal of Nursing Education* **46**(7): 299–303.

Newman TB (2003) The power of stories over statistics. *British Medical Journal* **327**: 1429–34

Petersen SK, Tribler J, Molsted S (2008) Empowerment – inspired patient education in practice and theory. *European Diabetes Nursing* **5**(3): 99–103

Petersson P, Springett J, Blomgvist K (2009) Telling stories from everyday practice, an opportunity to see a bigger picture; a participatory action research project about developing discharge planning. *Health and Social Care in the Community* **17**(6): 548–56

Rittman M, Stella S (1995) Storytelling. An innovative approach to story development. *Journal of Nursing Staff Development* **11**(1): 15–19

Schreiber R, Banister E (2002) Challenges of teaching in an emancipatory curriculum. *Journal of Nursing Education* **41**(1): 41–5

Spouse J (2003) *Professional learning in nursing.* Blackwell Publishers, Oxford

Starbuck D (2006) *Creative teaching: Getting it right.* Continuum, London.

Steen C, Costello J (2008) Teaching pre-registration nurse to assess acutely ill patients: An evaluation of an acute illness management programme. *Nurse Education in Practice* **8**: 343–51

Van Manen M (1990) *Researching lived experience: Human science for an action sensitive pedagogy.* Althouse Press, Ontario

Chapter 8

Empowered teams: Strength through positivity

Tony Ghaye

Introduction

Empowerment is an art. The art of knowing where and how to begin to build and then sustain empowered healthcare teams. This raises many questions. Some are about the culture of the workplace; others about relationships and communication, involvement and engagement. Yet more are about the timing and nature of critical actions and decisions. Arguably it is far better to make the right decisions slowly than the wrong decisions quickly. It is important to link actions with time for reflection upon them. Empowerment is also about values. It is about treating people in an appreciative way. Acknowledging that they have hopes and fears, their own aspirations and lives outside the workplace. It is also about treating them with respect and enabling them to feel that their views are heeded, that their talents are recognised and strengths used. Empowered teams are based on the notion that if we create the 'right' conditions, people can be trusted to do their best for the organisation. In doing so, there is a positive impact on organisational performance. Additionally it might not be helpful to think of empowerment in absolute terms. It is not black and white. It may be more appropriate to think of it in terms of how far you feel empowered. Is there any such thing, in the fast moving and ever changing world of health services, as being totally empowered or totally disempowered? Fundamentally, when teams within healthcare organisations move from more hierarchical, or command and control cultures, to more empowering ones, there is a shift in the power matrix. Some may feel a loss of power and that they have less control; others may feel advantaged, more positive and stronger.

So, in what ways do you feel you are valued and respected where you work? How far do you feel sufficiently resilient and therefore able to take knocks and set-backs? How many of your colleagues suffer from stress and are feeling burnt out? And above all, what strengthens you and what weakens you at work? What does your organisation do to attract 'great' people into its workforce? To what extent are you losing your best people? How far does your organisation set out to be the 'employer of choice' in managing and delivering healthcare services? All of these questions have an underlying thread. Arguably they are linked with aspects of empowerment. Empowerment is a term that is used repeatedly in health policy and practice in the UK. Currently it is often used in the context of empowering patients to make more informed decisions and particularly with staff engagement. Additionally, the more recent movements around the 'right to request', the starting up of social enterprises, employee-owned organisations, clinical autonomy and foundations trusts can all be seen as opportunities for feeling and becoming more empowered. These movements are all being linked with patient experience (e.g. dignity and privacy) and organisational performance. What we still do not know enough about is the nature and the flow of influence between processes of empowerment, patient experience, staff engagement and organisational performance.

The expansiveness of this word empowerment has been explored in this book. In general it has been conceived as both a process and an outcome. In this chapter I wish to make the case that empowered healthcare teams, of whatever kind, are strength-based teams. I see empowerment as a strength-based process and 'being empowered' as feeling strong and not weakened by the demands of our daily work. Another way of expressing this is that empowered teams contribute to, and are a result of, individual well-being. This implies a mindset shift away from teambuilding strategies that seek to empower teams by working on and getting rid of their 'problems' and more towards the identification, use and amplification of strengths. This is harder than it might seem. If we achieve it, we may make a significant contribution to reducing depression, enabling people to do better at work, to stay healthier, to become more resilient and even to live longer. This view of empowerment that I am advocating is linked with contemporary notions of human flourishing. It is a conscious effort to positively embrace human potentialities.

In the context of developing empowered healthcare teams I suggest that we need to ask three fundamental and practical questions:

- How far do people feel empowered?
- How has this happened?
- What can you do when you feel empowered that you could not do when you were experiencing feelings of disempowerment?

Talk of empowerment in healthcare has been fashionable for some time. Throughout much of the literature on empowerment there is an assumption that it is a 'good thing'. Some argue that it is better to be empowered than disempowered. But do staff and service users want to feel more empowered? What assumptions are we making here? Some say that being empowered is about being more effective, productive, fulfilled and healthier. When associated with the individual, empowerment is often called 'self-empowerment'. This term is linked to ideas of self-care, self-responsibility, self-determination, and personal control. It is to do with individuals taking control of their circumstances, achieving their personal desires and goals and trying to enhance the quality of their lives (Ghaye, 2005). But this chapter goes beyond individualism and focuses on some of the attributes and processes that lead to the formation of empowered teams.

In *Chapter 1* I argued that one enduring problem with empowerment is that it is often seen as a commodity, bestowed on those without it, by those who have it to give. It is a commodity that is given or withheld. If you have it, you are empowered. If not, then you are disempowered. This is a crude and simplistic view, linked to the consumer movement in healthcare in the 1980s and 90s. If empowerment is seen as something bestowed on healthcare staff and their patients/clients by those people who have it to give, rather than as something personally acquired through struggle and negotiation, then it might be better to regard it as just another form of social control or oppression (Ghaye 2011). It might be more helpful to regard empowerment as a process where, for instance, staff teams transform themselves in some beneficial manner. This usually involves some commitment to a 'cause', a group of patients/clients, or to a vision. The actual process can involve certain strategies or steps. These again can be problematic. For example, some describe this as a 'pass-it-on' process. This finds expression thus, 'Nurses themselves must first be empowered in order to be able to empower others' (Latter 1998: 24). Another example is the 'give-it-away' process. Again, this finds expression in such phrases as, 'We have to relinquish power, our role as expert, and pass control over to others'. This, of course, is potentially threatening for both parties. We can also find evidence of empowerment described as an 'enablement' process. This view asserts that the process is not so much about giving power away, as about creating opportunities which enable and encourage power to be taken.

In this chapter I explore four positive 'influencers' that contribute to the process of empowering teams. They are:

- Using positive emotions.
- Playing to your strengths.
- Ensuring that work is perceived as having meaning and purpose.
- Engaging positively with others within and outside the team.

These influencers are shown in *Figure 8.1*.

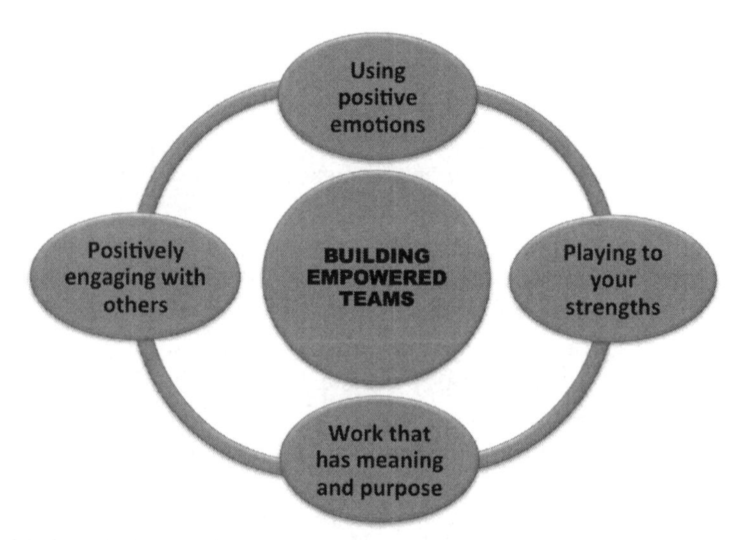

Figure 8.1. Some 'influencers' in building more empowered teams.

Using positive emotions: Positivity

Using positive emotions might be a good place to start an empowerment process. When motivating someone, or a team, it is good to focus on the positives, more than on weaknesses. When, in positive psychology, we talk about positive emotions we refer to emotions such as joy, gratitude, interest, hope, pride, inspiration and love. It is useful to use positive questions when trying to tap into the positive emotions that are 'there', or lie buried within us and get under-used and unappreciated because of the busyness of work. Positive questions can trigger positive conversations. Examples of positive trigger questions are:

- Think about a really positive experience for you when you felt appreciated and respected at work. What contributed to this?
- Think about a really positive experience for you when you felt you were able to cope well with your work. What contributed to this?
- Think about a really positive experience for you when you felt different ways of doing things were valued. What contributed to this?
- Which part of your job are you most passionate about and why?
- What were you doing when you had the greatest success or fulfilment in the last six months?

Table 8.1 sets out more trigger questions that might help elevate positive

Table 8.1. Trigger questions to elicit positive emotions in your team
Reflect upon, then try to create some time to talk about experiences that evoke JOY
• When have you felt safe, relaxed and joyful, glad about what was happening at that moment in your team? • When have things really gone your way, perhaps even better than expected?
Reflect upon experiences that evoke GRATITUDE
• When have you felt grateful or thankful, deeply appreciative of someone or something in your team? • When has someone gone out of their way to do something good for you?
Reflect upon experiences that evoke CALMNESS
• When have you felt fully at peace, truly content when working with colleagues? • When does your body feel completely relaxed, with all your physical tensions melted away?
Reflect upon experiences that evoke INTEREST
• When have you felt intensely open and alive in your teamworking, as you concentrate on something that fascinates you? • When have you felt an intense desire to explore and learn more about something of real interest to you?
Reflect upon experiences that evoke HOPE
• When have you felt hopeful and optimistic, encouraged by the possibilities of something good happening? • When have you been faced with uncertainty, but still somehow believed that things would change for the better?
Reflect upon experiences that evoke PRIDE
• When have you felt most proud of yourself and your team's achievements? • When have you achieved something great through your own efforts?
Reflect upon experiences that evoke INSPIRATION
• What has caused you to make even more effort to achieve something you never thought you could? • When have you seen someone in your team perform, or act, better than you ever imagined possible?
Reflect upon experiences that evoke LOVE
• When do you most readily feel the warmth of love between you and your colleagues? • When does a relationship of yours, with a colleague, evoke one of the other forms of positivity above?

emotions within your team. Conversations that are triggered by questions such as these are fundamentally emotional ones, so it is wise to check out how far those in your team are ready for them. What do you need to hang onto to enjoy such conversations? What needs to change for you to ask them? How unusual would it be to elevate positive emotions within your team by using phrases such as:

- This thrills me.
- I love this.
- I can't wait to ...
- I get so excited by ...

This might mean kicking the habit of conversations that include phrases, such as:

- I can't stand it when ...
- What really annoys me is ...
- I get frustrated when ...
- I'm so bored by ...

Using positive emotions to build a process of empowerment depends on how you think. Like all emotions, positive ones arise from the way you interpret ideas, actions and events as they unfold. How far are you aware that you have the power to turn positivity on and off for yourself?

Experiment with this. Turn positivity *on* right now. Ask yourself:

- What's right about my current circumstances?
- What makes me lucky to be in this team?
- What aspect of my current circumstances is a gift to be treasured?

Now turn positivity *off*. Ask yourself these positivity-spoiling questions:

- What's wrong with this team, right now?
- Why do I feel so fed up?
- Who can I blame for this?

Fredrickson (2001) and Fredrickson and Joiner (2002) talk about the power of positivity and the use of positive emotions. Fredrickson's (2001) broaden-and-build theory describes the form and function of a number of positive emotions, including joy, interest, contentment and love. A key idea within this theory is that these positive emotions broaden our thought–action repertoire. This means when we feel positive, we are generally more open-minded, more receptive to new ideas, more adaptive and more flexible. We feel stronger, more empowered to act. For example, joy sparks the urge to play, interest sparks the urge to explore, pride sparks the recurring cycle of trying to do the best job we can, each day. The broadened mindsets arising from these positive emotions are contrasted to the narrowed mindsets sparked by many negative emotions (i.e. specific action tendencies, such as to attack or flee). In other words when we feel more negative we feel much less prepared and able to consider alternatives, to 'play' with ideas and to consider options. We feel weakened. We may also feel disempowered. A second key idea of this theory is about the consequences of our broadened mindset. By broadening our thought–action repertoire, whether through play, exploration or similar activities, positive emotions promote discovery of novel and creative actions, ideas and social bonds, which in turn build our personal resources and ability to be resilient. These can range from physical and intellectual resources, to social and psychological ones. Importantly, these resources function as reserves that we can draw on later to improve the prospect of successful coping, survival, good work and good health. There is an important knock-on effect going on here. As positivity grows, so does our ability to be more open-minded and wholehearted in what we do. With this positive mindset comes a greater ability actually to try things out, to experiment and to improve what we do. Fredrickson (2009) argues that we can actually work at increasing our sense of positivity and that it also:

- Makes us feel good.
- Changes how our mind works.
- Can transform our future.
- Puts the brakes on negativity.

More specifically Fredrickson (2004: 1367) argues that,

> *... positive emotions signal optimal functioning, but this is far from their whole story .... positive emotions also produce optimal functioning, not just within the present, pleasant moment, but over the long term as well. The bottom-line message is that people should cultivate positive emotions in themselves and in those around them.*

Positivity is linked with self-regard. This means how a team sees itself. Self-regard is linked with self-esteem, which in turn is associated with feelings of self-worth. Self-efficacy is another important part of building a more empowered team. It relates to the team's belief in its ability to achieve its aims. So feeling empowered goes hand-in-hand with feelings of self-worth and self-regard. Without these, most teams struggle to find the necessary confidence and drive to bounce back from challenging situations and to be the best that they can each working day. Self-esteem is also associated with having a sense of perspective, which counteracts the tendency for paranoid thinking to develop (e.g. 'Why is it that this only happens to us?'). It also supports the process of bouncing back (e.g. 'What are we going to do to make this situation better next time?'). Self-esteem and high self-regard can help teams be more resilient. Empowered teams are resilient ones.

So, why is self-efficacy important when it comes to building empowered teams? Teams with high self-efficacy are more likely to be excited by challenges and view difficult tasks or situations as diversions rather than roadblocks. They are not knocked off course easily. Undaunted by the unknown, they take a broad view of the task in hand, in order to establish the best way forward. And they demonstrate significant tenacity in dealing with problems. Teams with low self-efficacy, on the other hand, assume that tasks are harder than they are. They worry about encountering failure rather than focusing on achieving success. They may prepare thoroughly, but since they tend to take a narrow (and sometimes short-sighted) view of a challenge, their planning is not always focused on the right priorities (Clarke and Nicholson 2010).

Positivity, as I am describing it, can be seen as a strength and ties in with my suggestion that empowered teams are strong teams. Positivity is also linked with job satisfaction. When we use our strengths in our job, most of the time, it is not surprising that we feel more positive about our work. We tend to get more pleasure from it and find it more meaningful. So two key reflective questions become:

- What percentage of last week did your team spend doing things that they really liked doing?
- What percentage of last week did your team spend playing to their strengths?

Answering these two questions means that you have been able to identify how, and where, particular strengths, that you feel your team has, are used in your current work. If you draw a blank over this you may wish to reflect upon these questions:

- How far are there missed opportunities, in your team, where you could, in different circumstances, spend more time using particular strengths?
- What new situations can your team put themselves in, so that they use the strengths that they possess?
- How could your team expand its current role to make better use of particular strengths?

Playing to your strengths

Conventional wisdom tells us that we learn from our mistakes, that we get better by fixing our weaknesses, by getting rid of what we do not want. Ask the people you work with point-blank, 'Is finding your weaknesses and fixing them the best way to achieve outstanding team performance?' Remember, the most useful definition of a weakness is an activity that makes you feel weak. It is an activity that, no matter how proficient you may (or may not) be at it, consistently produces negative emotional reactions. How does it serve you to believe that you will grow the most in your areas of greatest weakness?

The strengths movement, as it is now called, embraces the radical idea that all we learn from reflecting on our weaknesses is the characteristics of weaknesses. If we wish to learn about strengths we must study strengths. If we want to learn about successes, we must study success (Buckingham, 2007, Buckingham and Coffman 2005). If we want to know what constitutes 'good' (practices) then we must study them, not study bad practices. Why is it that we have a tendency to focus upon poor patient experiences when what we want are positive ones? Why do we tend to focus on disgruntled and demoralised team members to learn how to engage positively with them? Why do we run anti-bullying workshops when what we want is to learn about how staff can feel more valued and respected? Why do we study depression, narcosis and psychosis to learn about joy? We need a change in mindset. To build empowered teams, we need to study empowerment and learn more about how they have become that way.

If empowered teams are strong teams, we need to ask, what is a strength and what strengths do you have? It is not as easy as it may seem to define a strength. Is it about what we do best and/or what we do better than other people? The startling fact is that most of us do not know our strengths. We cannot list them easily. We do not know how many we have. We often get embarrassed when invited to talk about them. But we are acutely aware of our weaknesses. Kaiser (2009) argues that we need to be clear about how we define a strength. Most simply stated, strengths might be those talents, skills, and competencies a team has. But there is more to defining strengths than this. For example, we could look at strengths in at least two more ways. One is what measurement experts call an ipsative way. This refers to what the team is best at, independent of how good the team is compared to other teams. The second way to look at strengths is to compare your team's strengths to relevant and other teams. This is often called a 'normative' comparison because it considers how strong you are relative to an appropriate norm group, for example those doing similar kinds of work in community healthcare, in district nursing, podiatry, rehabilitation or care of the elderly.

What we can take away from these definitions is that if you feel that empowerment is indeed linked to the suggestion that it reflects an ability of a team to play to its strengths, then it would be prudent to try to make sure the team does more than just discover its strengths. Teams have to engineer occasions when they use these strengths as much as possible and develop new ones when necessary. In times of service re-organisation, for example, it is important for teams to develop and use strengths that enable them to stand out compared to other teams (competitive strengths).

What do you think will help you to be most successful in your work and to get most fulfilment from it? Building your strengths or fixing your weaknesses? Maybe it is a bit of both? If you gave these choices to members of your team, what do you think they would say? Working in target-driven, high performance-oriented, externally assessed and inspected NHS organisations, where resources are becoming scarcer, I think I know that they would suggest fixing their weaknesses. Maybe also, they would suggest using reflective practices to get rid of the things they do not do well and hopefully things will get better. When people use the cliché, 'people are our greatest assets', they do not mean that. They mean people's strengths are their greatest asset.

There has been much talk in the UK NHS about talent management. This is essentially making sure you have the right person in the right place at the right time. So NHS organisations have to work to ensure they are attracting, retaining and developing the right people to meet upcoming challenges. There is not much point in engaging new and talented people, who are also expensive, and then getting them positions in the organisation where they do not play to their strengths. How often do you feel your team plays to its strengths? Once a week? How would you all move from once a week to most of the time? Think a moment about the most successful and most fulfilled people you know, or work with. How much time do they spend using their strengths? Do they seem to spend most of their time doing activities that invigorate them? If you have anybody in mind, it may be prudent to reflect on the fact that what they do does not happen by accident. More realistically it happened because incrementally, week by week, somehow they managed to make the best of their job, into most of their job. So I am suggesting that we try to work out a way where reflective practices are used to deliberately tilt the world towards the best of you and your team, so that you can be the best you can, most of the time. Empowered teams build their work around their strengths. This does not mean they ignore their weaknesses. It means they are able to see their weaknesses in different ways and tackle them more creatively, from a position of strength. This feeling of empowerment enables us to reframe problems and challenges. Unfortunately, an obstacle stands in the way of enabling teams to positively embrace and develop their strengths. It is the negative attitude some have about hearing good news. Many of us are impatient with affirmation, with positive feedback and with compliments. Some regard this as simply a feel-good experience. It is criticism that is truly useful. It is the sting of failure that motivates us. It is reflecting on problems, and getting rid of them, that is the serious work to be done (Ghaye 2011). In *Table 8.2* there are a series of 10 questions that your team might find helpful in order to discover and talk about its strengths. Try completing them alone and then share your results with a colleagues.

Table 8.2. Discovering your strengths

Strength statement	*Response*
A major strength of mine is …	
When I get to use this strength I am specifically …	
When I am doing an activity that strengthens (not weakens) me I *feel* …	
When I am doing an activity that strengthens (not weakens) me I *think* …	
When I am doing an activity that strengthens (not weakens) me *I want to* …	
What *feedback*, if any, have you received about your strengths?	
What needs to change to enable you to use your strengths more often?	
What needs to change to enable those you work with, to use their strengths more often?	
What needs to change to enable those in your organisation, to use their strengths more often?	
How could you measure/track how much you use your strengths?	

Source: Ghaye, 2011

Ensuring that work is perceived as having meaning and purpose

Empowered teams are not preoccupied with thinking about what may be going wrong or what they are less pleased with. They are able to balance this with thoughts and conversations about what is going right and what they are happy with. Of course, sometimes it makes good sense to reflect upon problems and adverse events so that we can learn from them and avoid them happening again in the future. But if teams get into the habit of spending more time thinking about what is bad than good in their working lives, it can set team members up for anxiety and depression. Seligman (2011: 168–9) puts this in a powerful way.

> *We are bad-weather animals, naturally attracted to the most catastrophic interpretation of adversity, since we are the descendants of people who survived the Ice Age. Those of our ancestors who thought, 'It's a nice day in New York today; I bet it will be nice tomorrow', got crushed by the ice. Those who thought, 'It only looks like a nice day; here comes the ice, the flood, famine, the invaders, oy! Better store some food!' survived and passed down their brains to us. Sometimes thinking and planning for the very worst is useful; more often, however, it is paralysing and unrealistic.*

One way to keep this from happening is to get better at thinking about, and savouring, what went well. In order to do this, teams need to make sure that, for most of the time, their work has meaning and purpose. When I use these two terms I am referring to something that can be expressed thus; I generally feel that what I do at work and in my life is valuable and worthwhile. I suggest that work having meaning and purpose are two essential parts of becoming an empowered team. Work that is perceived as having meaning and purpose enhances well-being and employee engagement (Robertson Cooper, 2008). Without these two additional elements, any empowerment process is likely to falter.

Seligman (2011) has developed what he calls a What-Went-Well Exercise (also called 'Three Blessings'). It is a very useful exercise for teams to try. It is a way of checking out the extent to which team members have shared meanings about events and can agree on purposes. The first step is to write down three things that went well today at work. This can be done in a personal reflective journal or on a computer. It is important that everyone has a physical record of what they write so that they can reflect again on it in the light of step two. The three things need to be carefully selected. A criterion for selection is that they may be regarded as significant in some way. The second step is to answer the question, 'Why did this happen?', next to each significant event. The third step is to share events and their interpretation with others in the team. What is seen as a significant event?

Table 8.3 is a more elaborate and somewhat different approach to addressing meaning and purpose at work. It is a table of questions that can serve to generate a positive conversation about these two things. It is based upon the idea that if we change the question, we have a chance to change the conversation. Do this and we give ourselves an opportunity to change the action. The table also explicitly links meaning and purpose from within the individual, through teams and across whole organisations.

Table 8.3. Generating meaning and purpose from individuals through teams and across whole organisations

Main focus	*The individual*	*The work group or team*	*The whole organisation*
What's successful... right now? (*Appreciate*)	What do you feel you do really well and why?	What are your team's talents and achievements? How can you play to your strengths?	What are your organisation's major success stories? How can you contribute to them?
What do we need to change to make a better future? (*Imagine*)	What are some of your possibilities for improvement?	How can you ask appreciative questions to develop more strengths-based conversations amongst team members?	What options and alternatives do you have to increase performance and/ or productivity?
How do we do this? (*Design*)	What are your core values? Why do you hold these?	What are your team's values? Why do you hold these?	What are your organisation's values? What does it stand for?
Who takes action and with what consequences? (*Act*)	How far are you able to put your values into action?	How can you create more opportunities to do what you do best, every day?	How far is your performance aligned with mission?

Source : Ghaye (2011)

In a very practical way the following four questions about 'mattering' can aid our personal and collective understandings about meaning and purpose. They are:

- Does it matter why I/we do this activity?
- Does it matter who I/we do this activity with/to/for?
- Does it matter when I am/we are doing this activity?
- Does it matter what this activity is about?

A sense of purpose can be enhanced if a team, or NHS organisation, has realistic job previews in order to maximise the fit between the hopes and ambitions of individuals and the goals and mission of the organisation. Meaningful goal-setting, developing mutual understanding, shared values and the co-creation of ethos, can all enhance meaning and purpose at work.

Engaging positively with others within and outside the team

Empowerment is a complex process. In UK NHS organisations a much more strategic approach is increasingly needed if empowerment efforts are to be successful and sustainable. Arguably this requires the coordinated involvement of the organisation's Health and Safety, Occupational Health, Human Resources, Organisational Development, Patient and Liaison Services, Communications and other departments. Engagement can also be seen at a more micro level. For example, it can mean when an individual or team is absorbed in a task and time flies by. Engagement is an important part of an empowerment process. Arguably very little that is positive is solitary. Seligman (2011:20) puts it this way:

> *When was the last time you laughed uproariously? The last time you felt indescribable joy? The last time you sensed profound meaning and purpose? The last time you felt enormously proud of an accomplishment? Even without knowing the particulars of these high points of your life, I know their form: all of them took place around other people.*

When I suggest that engagement is a crucial part of any empowerment process, I am talking about the importance of positive relationships that serve to be a source of enrichment, vitality and learning for individuals, teams and organisations. So I have in mind a view of engagement that is far more than merely 'getting along with others' and avoiding arguments. Positively engaging with others brings with it many benefits. Cameron (2008: 41) puts it this way:

> *The most common assumption is that when people receive love, support and encouragement, when their psychological and emotional needs are met, they tend to feel secure, and their performance is therefore elevated. What has actually been found however, is that it is what people give to a relationship rather than what they receive from a relationship that accounts for the positive effects...The demonstration of altruism, compassion, forgiveness and kindness all were found to be necessary for positive relationships to have their maximum positive impact on well-being and performance.*

In 2009, NHS Employers published their improving staff engagement toolkit. Their list of key points can be read in many ways. Given what has been set out in this book this list of points looks like a list of things that both contribute to, and require, a more empowered workforce. The key points are:

- Engaged staff are more productive, less prone to absenteeism, better at engaging customers and less likely to leave.
- Investing the extra time in getting the right people into the right jobs from the start is essential.
- It is impossible to deny the business imperative of incorporating engagement initiatives into operating plans.
- There is growing evidence of a link between engaged staff and the quality of patient care and satisfaction.
- Improving engagement does not have to cost more and may actually save money.
- Managers play a significant role in influencing employee job performance and engagement levels.

A more recent publication, coordinated by the Care Quality Commission, called the NHS Staff Survey allows NHS employers to monitor the experiences of their staff. The results of the 2010 survey were published 2011. The section on staff engagement makes difficult reading. For example, it reports that staff motivation at work has declined. Additionally, although it states that there has been a small increase in staff reporting that they are able to suggest new ideas, there are no improvements in levels of staff involvement in decision making. Less than a third in the survey felt that senior managers acted on feedback from staff. This is sad because only by involving staff in decisions and communicating clearly with them, can trusts seek to maintain staff morale during this period of major change for the NHS. This is a rather gloomy picture of corrosive disempowerment.

It is not rocket science to appreciate that to feel empowered, staff need resources to do their work. These might be in the form of appropriate training or equipment. They need to be well-informed via good communication. Nothing is more disempowering than feeling that you are left out of the loop or that you are not able to keep in touch with important developments. Empowered teams are those that feel they can influence the way in which their work is organised. There is a real feeling that they are in control of things. One important challenge is to create opportunities for teams to become sources of positive energy and form positive energy networks with others, inside and beyond the organisation. Positive energisers create and support the vitality of others. They strengthen others. Collectively they play a vital part in becoming an empowered team.

References

Buckingham M (2007) *Go put your strengths to work: Six powerful steps to achieve outstanding performance.* Simon & Schuster, London

Buckingham M, Coffman C (2005) *First, break all the rules: What the world's greatest manager's do differently.* Pocket Books, London

Cameron K (2008) *Positive leadership: Strategies for extraordinary performance.* Berrett-Koehler, San Francisco, CA

Care Quality Commission (2011) *NHS staff survey results.* Department of Health, London

Clarke J, Nicholson J (2010) *Resilience: Bounce back from whatever life throws at you.* Crimson Publishing, Richmond, Surrey

Fredrickson B (2009) *Positivity: Groundbreaking research reveals how to embrace the hidden strength of positive emotions, overcome negativity, and thrive.* Crown Publications, New York

Fredrickson B (2004). The broaden-and-build theory of positive emotions. *Philosophical Transactions of the Royal Society* **359**: 1367–78.

Fredrickson B (2001) The role of positive emotions in positive psychology: The broaden-and-build theory of positive emotions. *American Psychologist* **56**(3): 218–226

Fredrickson B, Joiner T (2002) Positive emotions trigger upward spirals toward emotional well-being, *Psychological Science* **13**(2): 172–5

Ghaye T (2005) *Developing the reflective healthcare team.* Blackwell Publishing, Oxford

Ghaye T (2011) *Teaching and learning through reflective practice: A practical guide for positive action* (2nd edn). Routledge, Abingdon, Oxford

Kaiser RB (2009) *The perils of accentuating the positive.* Hogan Press, Tulsa, OK

Latter S (1998) Health promotion in the acute setting: The case of empowering nurses. In S Kendall (ed) *Health and empowerment: Research and practice*. Arnold, London

NHS Employers (2009) *Briefing 68. Improving staff engagement: A practical toolkit.* NHS Employers, London

Robertson Cooper (2008) *Well-being at work: The new view.* Robertson Cooper, Manchester

Seligman MEP (2011) *Flourish: A visionary new understanding of happiness and well-being*. Free Press, New York

Index

A

advance
  care plans 111–112
  decisions 112
  directives 112
  statements 111–112
ageing
  and empowerment 67–68
  and intelligence 70–71
  and personality 74–75
  and self-image 73–74
  defining 69–70
  social 71–72
assault
  on nurses 50–53
autonomy 40–43

B

best interests
  of patients 113–114

C

caring
  role of nurses 30
  value-based 30
Children and Young People's Project (2009–2010) 91–94
commissioning
  involvement of young people in 84
communication
  barriers to 110
  between staff and patients 109
conscientisation 15
Convention on the Rights of the Child 80–81
conversations
  difficult 109

D

decision making
  ethical 31

E

emotions
  use of positive 132
empowered teams
  influencers 132, 150
empowerment 6
  and best interests of the patient 113–114
  and power 12
  and reversals in power 17
  as a commodity 10
  as a discourse 13
  as a process 11
  as a way of thinking 11
  as developing a voice 12
  as personal reality 14
  collective 10
  for older people 65
  healthcare practitioners' role 114
  inter-personal 84
  intra-personal 85
  of children and young people 84–85
  of students 119–120, 123
  of the individual 9–10
  psychological 85
  roots of 14
  stages of 11
  through storytelling 121–122
  understanding of 8

end of life care
decisions about 110–111
End of Life Care Strategy 108
environment
effect on violence 56
ethical
decision making 31
barriers to 37
nurses' role in 35
decisions
strategies 36
reflection 42–44
ethics 30
and nursing interaction 38–40
as dilemma in healthcare 32–33
nurses' stories 38–41
points for reflection 45
evidence-based practice 7

F

Freire, Paulo 15, 16, 17, 109

H

hypothetico-deductive approach 21

I

Independent Complaints Advocacy Services 82–83

J

job satisfaction 136

L

lasting power of attorney 113
living will 112

M

meaning and purpose of work 140

N

National End of Life Programme 114
National Service Frameworks 28
Nursing and Midwifery Code of Conduct 37

P

palliative care 107
participation 80–81
of children and young people 87–88
Patient Advice and Liaison Services 82–83
patient and public involvement 82–83
positive engagement 142
positivity 132–134
power 19
over, with, to and within 100
prediction
of aggressive behaviour 58
Public Inquiries 28
purpose 140

R

reflective practices
and enhancement of professional development 6
and improvement of clinical environment 7
and power relationships 6
an quality of care 5
appeal of 3
current claims for 5–7
right
to be heard 90
to express views 90
to respect for views 90
rights
of children and young peole 89–90
role-play 94–97

S

self-efficacy 136
self-empowerment 9, 67, 131
self-image
 and ageing 73–74
Standards and Care Benchmarks 28
storyboarding 122–123
 and narrative 120–121
 empowering students through 123
 history of 120
storytelling
 to empower students 121–122
strengths
 of the team 137

T

team
 empowerment of 132, 150
 strengths and weaknesses of 137
theories-of-action 8

V

violence
 against nurses 52
 effects of environment 56
 prediction of 55, 58

W

weaknesses
 of teams 137